Dr. R[...] [...]
to
Talking about Herpes

ALSO BY DR. RUTH K. WESTHEIMER

Musically Speaking: A Life Through Song

Conquering the Rapids of Life: Making the Most of Midlife Opportunities
with Pierre A. Lehu

The Lover's Companion: Art and Poetry of Desire edited by Charles Sullivan

Human Sexuality: A Psychosocial Approach with Dr. Sanford Lopater

Who am I? Where Did I Come From? with Pierre A. Lehu

Dr. Ruth, Grandma on Wheels with Pierre A. Lehu

Power: The Ultimate Aphrodisiac with Dr. Steven Kaplan

Rekindling Romance for Dummies with Pierre A. Lehu

Dr. Ruth's Guide to College Life with Pierre A. Lehu

Dr. Ruth's Pregnancy Guide for Couples with Amos Grunebaum, M.D.

Grandparenthood with Dr. Steven Kaplan

Dr. Ruth Talks about Grandparents with Pierre A. Lehu

The Value of Family with Ben Yagoda

Heavenly Sex: Sex in the Jewish Tradition with Jonathan Mark

Sex for Dummies

Dr. Ruth's Encyclopedia of Sex

Dr. Ruth Talks to Kids

The Art of Arousal

Dr. Ruth's Guide to Safer Sex

Surviving Salvation, with Professor Steven Kaplan

Dr. Ruth's Guide to Sensuous and Erotic Pleasures with Dr. Louis Lieberman

Sex and Morality: Who Is Teaching Our Sex Standards?
with Dr. Louis Lieberman

All in a Lifetime

Guide to Married Lovers

First Love

Dr. Ruth's Guide to Good Sex

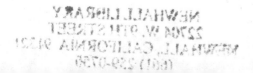

Dr. Ruth's Guide
to
Talking about Herpes

DR. RUTH K. WESTHEIMER
and Pierre A. Lehu

Grove Press
New York

Published simultaneously in Canada
Printed in the United States of America

FIRST EDITION

Library of Congress Cataloging-in-Publication Data

Westheimer, Ruth K. (Ruth Karola), 1928–
Dr. Ruth's guide to talking about herpes / Ruth K. Westheimer
and Pierre A. Lehu.
p. cm.
ISBN 0-8021-4120-X
1. Herpes genitalis. 2. Herpes genitalis—Treatment. I. Title: Doctor Ruth's
guide to talking about herpes. II. Lehu, Pierre A. III. Title.
RC203.H45W477 2004
616.95'18—dc22   2003064146

Grove Press
an imprint of Grove/Atlantic, Inc.
841 Broadway
New York, NY 10003

04 05 06 07 08   10 9 8 7 6 5 4 3 2 1

*To all those in the fields of medicine and
pharmacology who have toiled so hard against
herpes and every other disease that afflicts mankind.*

Contents

Medical Disclaimer

Dr. Ruth's Guide to Talking about Herpes is not intended to replace medical advice and should be used to supplement rather than replace regular care by your doctor. It is recommended that you seek your physician's advice before embarking on any medical program or treatment. All efforts have been made to ensure the accuracy of the information contained in this book as of the date of publication. The publisher and the authors disclaim liability for any medical outcomes that may arise as a result of applying the advice suggested in this book.

Privacy Disclaimer

The names of the individuals discussed in this book have been changed to protect their privacy.

Foreword

by Peter Anthony Leone, M.D.

At a recent conference with Dr. Ruth Westheimer, I stated, in the hope of relating we all are sexual beings, that sex was inevitable and that sex was a lot more like eating than smoking. Dr. Westheimer immediately stood up and said, "No, Peter, sex is BETTER than eating." She was right, and with one statement she was able to lighten the mood of a conference specifically focusing on genital herpes and drive home the point that sex can and should be great. More to the point of this book, sex can and should be great even after a diagnosis of genital herpes.

On any given day in America, there are more people living with genital herpes than infected with the common cold. True, over the course of a year there are more new infections with cold viruses than new genital infections with herpes simplex, but herpes lasts a lifetime. With an estimated sixty million adults with genital herpes and an additional one million new infections each year, why do we find it so difficult to talk about herpes and how can it be that so few of us know someone with herpes? The AIDS epidemic trivialized herpes in the imagination of the public. This, along with our inability

to talk comfortably about sex, marginalized the available information about herpes. Furthermore, the stigma associated with the diagnosis deters patients from pursuing a diagnosis. The medical
community is equally complicit, often avoiding a diagnosis that
neither patient nor doctor want to face. As a result, the herpes epidemic moves onward due to our complacent silence while causing
physical and psychological discomfort, devastating infections in
newborn infants, and the further expansion of the HIV pandemic.

During the past decade, I have provided medical care for people
living with genital herpes, and I have been trying to find a better
way to get the word out that this is a "common" disease. You need
not live an extraordinary life to either acquire it or to live with it.
In a way that only she can, Dr. Westheimer provides information
about the virus, the disease, and how to live with rather than suffer
with genital herpes. The medical information presented in this book
is a snapshot of where we are currently with herpes, but the stories
told by those infected with herpes are timeless. Dr. Westheimer has
spent over twenty years getting us to talk about sexuality, sex, and
its consequences with the same passion that we have for sex itself.
Few teachers about the human condition have been willing to lend
their voices to any sexually transmitted disease other than HIV. Yet
Dr. Ruth Westheimer has never been afraid to talk about things
others would not discuss, and she is, above all else, an educator.
Knowledge is power and ignorance can only increase the risk of
acquiring or transmitting genital herpes. In this book, Dr.
Westheimer provides vital information about genital herpes. The
chapters of this book trace the steps of dealing with a diagnosis of
genital herpes and provide specific information for wherever one
may be in life. In these chapters are reflections by individuals
diagnosed with herpes. These stories are not meant to replace
accurate medical information, nor are they intended to mirror your
current life situation. But they may provide hope, present a template
for discussing herpes with those you love, and assuage the sense of

isolation that often follows diagnosis of a sexually transmitted disease.

There are no current cures for genital herpes and no absolute way to prevent transmission. The information and stories Dr. Westheimer relates in this book will certainly help. We need more champions for open discussions concerning sex and its consequences. Thank God for Dr. Ruth. Her warmth and care has given a safe opportunity for the heroes in this book to share their stories. In doing so, maybe, just maybe, we have moved one step closer to destigmatizing this most common of sexually transmitted diseases.

Acknowledgments

Dr. Ruth K. Westheimer's Acknowledgments:

To the memory of my entire family who perished during the Holocaust. To the memory of my late husband, Fred, who encouraged me in all my endeavors. To my current family, my daughter Miriam Westheimer, Ed.D., son-in-law Joel Einleger, M.B.A., their children Ari and Leora, my son Joel Westheimer, Ph.D., daughter-in-law Barabara Leckie, Ph.D., and their children Michal and Benjamin. I have the best grandchildren in the entire world!

Thanks to all the many family members and friends for adding so much to my life. I'd need an entire chapter to list them all but some must be mentioned here: Pierre Lehu and I have now collaborated on a dozen books, he's the best Minister of Communications I could have asked for! Dr. Peter Leone for teaching me so much about herpes and for his valuable contributions to this book, Cliff Rubin, my assistant, thanks! Ruch Bachrach, David Best, M.D., Daniel Buchbinder, M.D., Carlita C. de Chavez, Marcie Citron,

Martin Englisher, Cynthia Fuchs Epstein, Ph.D., Howard Epstein, David Goslin, Ph.D., Allan Halpern, M.D., Fred Howard, Vera Jelinek, Alfred Kaplan, Steve Kaplan, Ph.D., Amy Kassiola, Joel Kassiola, Ph.D., Bonnie Kaye, Richard and Barbara Kendall, Robert Krasner, M.D., Marga and Bill Kunreuther, Dean Stephen Lassonde, Rabbi and Mrs. William Lebeau, Mark Lebwohl, M.D., Lou Lieberman, Ph.D. and Mary Cuadrado, Ph.D., John and Ginger Lollos, William J. Maher, Dale Ordes, Robert Pinto, Philip Prioleau, M.D., Fred and Anne Rosenberg, Simeon and Rose Schreiber, Daniel Schwartz, Amir Shaviv, John and Marianne Slade, Betsy Sledge, William Sledge, M.D., Hannah Strauss, Jeff Tabak, Esq., Greg Willenborg, Ben Yagoda, and Froma Zeitlin, Ph.D. And to all of the people who worked so hard to bring this book into print at Grove Atlantic especially Eric Price and Brando Skyhorse. And finally to all those millions of people who have herpes, and in particular those special individuals who agreed to participate in the creation of this book; your contribution was invaluable.

Pierre A. Lehu's Acknowledgments:

Thanks to my wife, Joanne Seminara, children, Peter and Gabrielle, mother, Annette Lehu, in-laws, Joe and Anita Seminara, and all the Seminara clan. And I, too, must thank Dr. Peter Leone for answering our many questions so promptly and clearly, and the people with herpes who gave us their stories, which opened our eyes to the silver lining that often accompanies this widespread disease.

Thou shalt love thy neighbor as thyself
Leviticus 19:18

Talking about Herpes:
An Introduction

In 1980, when my New York radio show debuted, herpes had just hit the headlines; when the show went live a year later, many of the questions people asked me were about this surging sexually transmitted disease (STD). A short while later, AIDS was making headlines and herpes was relegated to the media doghouse. But while there's no denying that AIDS is a much more serious STD than herpes—for AIDS is a killer and herpes is not—herpes has done its share of damage, and today it is estimated that nearly 60 million Americans are infected with this disease.

It's possible that even if herpes had remained in the headlines it would have spread as broadly as it has, but I personally believe that as soon as herpes was demoted in the ranking of STDs, it caused people to lose much of their fear of being infected, creating ideal conditions for its widespread transmission.

Since I'm not a medical doctor, I'm afraid there's not much that I can do about the medical consequences of this epidemic. I will share whatever I've learned about herpes in the first chapter, and rest assured that an expert in the field has looked this material over so that it is completely accurate. But while I have a duty to tell you the basics about herpes in a book such as this, that is not my main purpose for writing it. In addition to the physical symptoms, herpes carries a lot of psychological baggage, and helping people deal with those issues is the main reason why I wanted to write a book about this disease.

Nathaniel Hawthorne wrote a novel called *The Scarlet Letter* in which the heroine is sentenced to wear a large scarlet *A* on her dress to denote that she is an adulteress. This may have been appropriate punishment in the seventeenth century, but today, no one is forced to reveal past sins to the general public in this way, including that one has been infected by a sexually transmitted disease. But for someone who has one of these diseases, and especially herpes, it can sometimes seem as if a large letter *H* is visible for all to see on their forehead; it is especially visible to any potential partners. That's because they know that at some point in a budding relationship, the truth will have to come out, and that dreaded moment can hang like the classic sword of Damocles over the head of the herpes sufferer. In some cases, the fear of having such a discussion, and the possible rejection that it might cause, is so strong that these individuals never date anyone ever again.

I've counseled people faced with this situation, so I know how much anguish it can cause. I will be giving advice and tips on how to handle this very touchy moment, based on the advice I've given to these clients. One advantage of being a therapist is that you get feedback on the advice you give so you know what works and what doesn't, and I hope you'll benefit from what I have to say. But I'm also going to give you more than simply my thoughts on the issue, since my practice doesn't have a regular flow of people with herpes. What you're also going to find in this book are excerpts from interviews with real people who have herpes and have had to tackle the various problems that having herpes causes.

These excerpts are scattered throughout the book and I believe you'll find them very useful.

The reason that reading such stories may be very important to you is that herpes is a disease that needs to be put into its proper perspective. It's not deadly, but it does have serious repercussions. Under normal circumstances, if you faced a heavy-duty problem, you'd be able to take some of the burden off of your shoulders by talking about it with family and friends. For example, if you were thinking of getting contact lenses, you probably know at least half a dozen people who wear them and could share their trials and tribulations. Or when someone you were dating was acting selfishly or boorishly, your friends would be there to give you advice. But even though there are some 60 million other people in similar shoes in this country, since herpes is not something you ordinarily drag into the conversation, there's no way of knowing which of your friends and acquaintances may have it—or would be willing to talk about it. And while there are support groups out there, they are few and far between, especially given the numbers of sufferers, so their meetings can be hard to find and even harder to attend. So with herpes, if you want advice from people who have been through what you're going through, a book such as this may be the only source.

Even if you know someone with herpes who is willing to talk about what happened to them, their advice might not be entirely useful. Their particular experience might not fit your circumstances. And if they pass on medical information, it might not be correct. But in these pages I'm going to give you an entire book full of stories, and not only will some quite likely be very similar to yours, but even those that aren't should provide you with some useful information. And I'll also be filling in these stories with my professional perspective, which will help you to get the most from them.

There was a bit of a master plan when organizing this book, but if you have a partner, for example, you may want to skip the chapter about finding a partner and go right to the one that deals with living with herpes as a couple. It's okay to jump around, but I would suggest that you read even the chapters that don't appear to apply to you. Remember, this book is supposed to help you deal with the psychological aspects of herpes, and since I think you'll benefit by reading all of the various things the people that were interviewed had to say, I believe it would be useful for you to read even the parts that don't appear to be relevant. You might find something said there that applies to your past, and since your past affects your current life and your future, any insights that you could get might prove very useful.

I wish that I could promise you that from reading this book, all your experiences with herpes are going to turn out to be positive ones. But I can't do that, for like most medical problems, herpes is a burden and there will be a price to pay for having caught it. This book won't cure you of herpes or make the issues it raises go away. What it can do is mitigate the effect that herpes will have on your life by teaching you how to best deal with those effects.

And let me end this introduction with my usual spiel, which is one that I believe in wholeheartedly: If having herpes is really bringing you down, consult with a mental health professional. Obviously you should see a medical doctor, if you haven't already done so, to deal with the physical symptoms. There are drugs that can help you and you need to know all you can about them. But if herpes is making you depressed or anxious, a mental health professional can help ease those types of symptoms. So if you feel that herpes is bringing you so low that it's ruining your life, don't just bottle up all these negative emotions, but instead pour them out to a counselor who has the experience to help you to cope.

1

Herpes, the Disease

While the virus that gives you genital herpes has been around for a long time, definitely centuries but quite possibly thousands of years, it's only for a few decades that the general public has been aware of it. Why this sudden stepping out into the spotlight? Clearly the sexual revolution made the spread of all sexually transmitted diseases grow by leaps and bounds, and since herpes was not widely known, and because there was no cure, it quickly became a "star." But as many celebrities who've tasted stardom can tell you, fame can be fleeting, and so almost as quickly as herpes stepped up onstage, it was knocked out of the limelight by AIDS. But just because herpes no longer gets top billing doesn't mean that it no longer poses a danger. Perhaps the fact that herpes has been lurking in the shadows for the last couple of decades is the main reason that it has spread so widely. As I already mentioned, it is believed that as many as 60 million people in the United States alone are infected with this virus, and it's also widespread all around the globe. What we're going to explore in this chapter are the consequences of this epidemic on the most basic level, in your life.

While many of those reading this book already have herpes, I'm going to assume that you don't know that much about this disease. That's an attitude I would suggest that you adopt as well, even if you think you have a good working knowledge of this scourge, because some of what you know might be wrong, and the consequences of any misinformation could be quite serious. In preparing this book, I've met with some of the top specialists in the world on herpes, so I might be able to pass on some information that you're not aware of, particularly if you've had herpes for some time and haven't done any further research recently.

A Caveat

While there is much that is known about herpes, I have to tell you right away that there is also a lot that is not known. That's not too surprising when you think that we haven't even found a cure for the common cold. It would be great if a doctor could wave some electronic gizmo over you, as they do on *Star Trek,* and cure you of whatever ails you, but while medical science has made some amazing leaps and bounds, it is still grounded by the limitations that exist today on planet Earth. So the bad news is that whatever we do know about herpes, there is still no cure, but the good news is that there are drugs that can help you, and I'll get to them a bit later on.

Two Types of Herpes

I did a duet on a CD of children's songs with Tom Chapin called *Two Kinds of Seagulls.* In it we sang (actually, Tom sang and I talked) about different pairs of animals (as in he-gulls and she-gulls). As it turns out, there are also two kinds of herpes. (If you want to get very technical, there are really eight, but there's no need to get quite so technical for our purposes other than to say that among the diseases these other herpes viruses cause are chicken pox, mononucleosis, and "sixth disease.") The two types of herpes virus we are concerned with in this book are herpes simplex virus 1 (HSV-1) and herpes simplex virus 2 (HSV-2). The main difference between the two is their choice of living quarters. HSV-1 prefers to reside in the upper half of your body and HSV-2 prefers the lower half. That's why HSV-1 is mostly responsible for cold sores and HSV-2 is responsible for genital herpes. (With oral sex so much more prevalent these days, some cases of genital herpes are actually HSV-1, while HSV-2 may be found in the mouth, but more on that later.)

I'm sure you've seen someone with a cold sore, if you haven't experienced one of these yourself, so you know what HSV-1 looks like when it is in its visible form. (In fact, 80 to 90 percent of Americans over the age of fifty are seropositive for HSV-1, meaning they've been infected at some point in their life with HSV-1.) On the other hand, if you don't have genital herpes, you may not have seen what it looks like, and I'm not going to show you in this book. If you have genital herpes, or if your partner has it, then you already know what the lesions herpes causes look like, so there's no real purpose in showing you images from other cases, especially as the ones that make the best photos are usually the worst cases. (Many are taken of people who have suppressed immune systems and so have the worst symptoms possible, much worse than average.) And even if you don't have herpes and have never seen a herpes lesion up close, I still don't want to fill your head with terrible pictures. I know that scare tactics don't work, at least when it comes to dousing a person's arousal when it's very strong, so there's no point in trying to scare my readers with gruesome pictures. And if you ever discover any sores, blisters, or lesions on either yourself or a partner, rather than playing guessing games and trying to decide what it may or may not be on your own by comparing your lesions to pictures in a book, I strongly suggest that the infected person go to see a doctor as quickly as possible to get the real answer. As you'll see later on, even doctors can misdiagnose it, so there's really no point in your trying to guess what caused whatever lesions you are seeing.

HSV-2 is called genital herpes because the visible signs appear as little bumps, blisters, or a rash in the genital area, thighs, or buttocks. Many people notice some itching, tingling, stinging, or even actual pain in the area before any visible signs are evident. This is called *prodome*.

But someone could also have caught herpes and never exhibit any visible signs at all. The fact is, 90 percent of people who have herpes don't know they have it. That's because either they had no symptoms of herpes at all, or only very minor indications and didn't recognize them as being a sign of herpes. A male might think that what he is seeing is nothing more than jock itch, while a female might feel some itching inside her vagina, but not think it serious enough to investigate further, chalking it up to a yeast infection.

The Initial Outbreak

Shannon—My first outbreak was terrible and lasted about a week. It hurt to pee, and it made me cry at times. I was covered in blisters in the genital area. After that, I seemed to get one or two blisters once or twice a month for a while, especially around my monthly cycle. They would burn or tingle just a bit at times, but they were more uncomfortable than bothersome. They'd last a few days and be gone. As time went by, the outbreaks got further apart. About once every three to six months I'd get a mild outbreak with one or two blisters that would last two to three days. Sometimes they would occur more often, sometimes less often. They seemed to occur the most often when I was under a lot of stress.

While it's true that 90 percent of people who get herpes don't know it, among those who do, the initial outbreak can be quite severe (and the first one is usually the most severe). When the herpes virus first penetrates the skin, it quickly begins to multiply. If symptoms are going to appear, they'll show up between two and twenty days afterward. Along with any blisters, the infected person may also feel pain, have flulike symptoms, get swollen lymph glands, and feel a burning sensation when urinating. The blisters will eventually break open and become sores, which can take from two to three weeks to heal. Certainly anyone with these types of symptoms should immediately visit a doctor. There may be no cure but there are medications that can alleviate the symptoms. Three drugs currently used are acyclovir, famciclovir, and valacyclovir. Check with your doctor as to what treatment would be appropriate for you to use.

I know that these days many medical products can be ordered over the Internet, basically without a prescription, and at a lower cost than at a drugstore. But because any drug may have side effects, please don't self-medicate. I'm not going to tell you where you should shop to fill a prescription—though you can't be as positive that a drug bought on the Web is really what it is said to be as you can when you go to your neighborhood pharmacy—but definitely start out by asking a doctor what you should be taking, and how often, and so on.

However, as I said, there needn't be any visible signs for a person to be infected—at least nothing that the human eye could detect. But the infection has still occurred, and the herpes virus is still capable of being passed on to someone else, who may then get a full-blown case with quite painful, recurring blisters. So if someone ever accuses you of having given them herpes, before you plead innocence, go have yourself tested. It's quite possible that you have it but just don't know it, which is why despite being a very moral individual, you didn't inform this partner or take any precautions, such as using a condom when having sex. You may not be to blame for any infections you caused before such an accusation, but if rather than getting tested, you ignore this current warning, then any further infections fall squarely on your shoulders. I'm going to give you more information on the moral issues revolving around telling potential partners about herpes later in this book.

The Latency Phase

After the initial infection the virus retreats to the spine, where it lives in the neurons. This is called the *latency phase*. Every once in a while—which could mean weeks, months, or maybe even years, though typically people get three to four outbreaks a year—the virus leaves its refuge and travels along the nerves to cause another outbreak. No one knows exactly what triggers such a migration, though it is believed that fever, intercurrent infection, and exposure to ultraviolet radiation (i.e., sunlight) can cause an outbreak of HSV-1. No such triggers have been identified for HSV-2; some laypeople believe that stress, menstruation, sexual activity, or diet may be triggers, but the medical world has found no scientific proof of this.

> **Mark**—Among those in the support groups, there are lots of reports of different causes. Diet and the menstrual cycle are two common ones. Many people find it's stress that causes an outbreak. Other things I've heard are abrasion, heavy-duty sex or masturbation, riding a bicycle for a long time, or exercising on a rowing machine. You have to know your own body. I suggest that you keep a diary so that you'll see patterns evolving and then you can discover what triggers you might have.

Because the immune system has gone to work as a result of the first attack, subsequent attacks tend to be less severe. In fact, the immune response to one type of herpes, say HSV-1, will cause an initial attack of the other form of herpes to be less severe, and may even act to prevent an infection of the other type of herpes altogether. (Notice that I said "may," so don't count on the fact that you have HSV-1 as guaranteeing you from ever getting HSV-2. Different studies have come up with different conclusions, so the real answer is still up in the air.)

As the years go by, there is usually a natural lessening of the yearly number of attacks. There are no exact statistics to offer you, and the rate of decline will depend on which type of herpes virus is causing the symptoms.

Moving Right Along

Meigan—I had about a three-year "remission" (if one can call it that) from outbreaks which had been occurring until that point on my outer labia, and along my inner groin area where the elastic of the panties would hit. I had had herpes for about six or seven years at this point, although I hadn't been diagnosed right away. Then one day I had a small dime-sized cluster of blisters in the middle of the right buttock area, about an inch or two to the left of a French-cut panty line. They would tingle, itch, and last about as long as most primary outbreaks, for about a week or so. Since I am fair-skinned, they would also leave my skin discolored pink, like a scar that is fading, for about a month.

Sometimes I would have one outbreak dissipating while another was beginning right next to it. These outbreaks were (pardon the pun) more of a pain in the butt than the genital ones had become, because it was like starting all over again: frequent outbreaks, lasting a week or ten days, more tingling and itching. The genital outbreaks had become infrequent—even as much as a three-year break—had become less tingly or itchy, and had even been coming up but not going "full-blown" (full-blown being watery blisters that pop), and then healing without becoming open sores (this is great because they are not as uncomfortable and heal faster). So, I was a little irritated that I was having herpes trouble again at such a rate, although, I did not have to worry about urine stinging the outbreak as sometimes happens with genital outbreaks (OBs).

As you can see from Meigan's case, when the herpes viruses leave their home in your spine and start roaming, they don't necessarily travel to the same place. So while it is more likely that a man who had his first attack of herpes on his penis will have subsequent attacks there, the blisters might also show up on his testicles, thigh, or buttocks. These viruses seem to have a mind of their own, so if there's one constant with herpes it's that you should expect the unexpected.

Since Meigan provided me with a lot of details that I feel could be helpful to others, let me quote some more of what she had to say about her outbreaks.

My doctor noticed the pink scarring on my buttocks when I went in for a checkup and suggested that since I was having more than six OBs a year I might do well to try an antiviral. At first I was only on OB therapy and wouldn't begin taking any medication until the first tingle. Only as soon as I would stop taking them I would have another outbreak, either in the exact same place or right next to it. So, I went on suppressive therapy, taking medication every day. That pretty much did the job. The buttocks OBs were really not much of an annoyance anymore. The only exceptions to that were times of extreme stress either brought on by work (I had been and still am a public elementary school teacher in schools of economically disadvantaged students), or newly married stresses. During those times I would have a "breakthrough outbreak" when the HSV in my system was wreaking havoc so much so that it overpowered the antiviral dosage in my system. However, the antiviral meds helped keep the outbreak from becoming too severe. Sometimes the skin would just turn pink and get sensitive and would not blister at all, and fade away in twenty-four hours.

By this time my greatest coping mechanism was Band-Aids. I would slap on two or three Band-Aids to cover the outbreak area completely. This seems to help keep me from wanting to scratch it (as inconspicuously as possible, of course). It was also kind of a relief to know the outbreak was not on my genitals, being a newlywed and all. Even though my husband had already contracted it, he never had another OB past the primary OB, so we remained "aware" of my OBs (mostly because I had Band-Aids on my butt) and were careful not to tempt fate by being careless during times of exposure, although we did not let it hinder our sex life together because it just became part of normalcy for us.

I do, on the rare occasion, get a genital outbreak. These are usually extremely tiny, not like the dime- to quarter-sized OBs on the buttocks. I might get a genital OB every two or three years. The buttocks OBs migrated from the right side to the left side after about two years, and now I'm susceptible to getting them on either side and even at the top of the crack of my buttocks or right above it.

As you can see from Meigan's experiences, there's really no telling when herpes will pay you a visit, or where.

Which HSV Is It?

Julie—It began with symptoms which I thought were related to a yeast infection but when the pain became horrible and with the combination of lesions, cuts, bumps, and all-over redness, I became pretty concerned. I was sure I had some awful flesh-eating virus and couldn't understand why it would start by attacking my vulva. I have been happily, monogamously married for eight years and we've been together for thirteen years and I just couldn't imagine herpes was the culprit, but all of my symptoms indicated a classic primary outbreak. By the time the doctor examined and cultured me, I had a pretty good idea what he would say. He said it looked pretty clear to him and started me on antivirals.

I found the Herpes Home Page (thank God, they were sooooo helpful) and posted many questions there. I did not yet have my culture and therefore my type back yet and there was a good amount of discussion about which type I likely had. After talking long and hard with my husband, I believe he has been faithful. He says he believes me. We both admitted that we had a little, tiny bit of doubt, but we were continuing to talk and we were just confused. Many people on the message board thought I might have been harboring this for many years and that the stress of my mother's recent death and all the illness I had been experiencing brought it to the surface. Others thought that maybe my husband had it without any symptoms and just passed it along to me.

I finally found out it is type 1 and things began to be clear to me. My husband has type 1 orally and gave it to me about twelve years ago. He had begun to feel a cold sore weeks prior to my outbreak, but it never materialized. It had been many days since he felt any tingling and we had oral sex. The fact that I already have the same strain orally made it confusing. I and others thought that I should have some antibodies to protect me — not from contracting HSV, but from having such a horrific outbreak. But I seem to be an exception to the general rule. The outbreak truly was worse than I would wish on my worst enemy (and I've given birth vaginally three times — I know pain down there)!

I am currently experiencing my second outbreak. It is uncomfortable, but *nothing* compared to the first. My husband and I have resumed our sex life and have found that other than during an outbreak, things have changed very little (though that first time was a little scary). Now I'm sure to wash with soap beforehand and he is sure to afterward.

As I mentioned earlier, while HSV-2 is more rarely seen as a cause of herpes sores in the oral cavity, and is almost always associated with an HSV-2 genital infection, HSV-1 does cause herpes in the genital region in a percentage of cases. This is undoubtedly a result of the increase of oral sex in the population. It is these cases of HSV-1 in the genital region, added to the HSV-2 genital infections, that cause experts to arrive at the figure of 60 million people with genital herpes.

While a case of genital herpes caused by HSV-1 is clinically no different from a case caused by HSV-2, the rate of recurrence is much less. While HSV-2 genital herpes usually recurs four times a year, genital herpes caused by HSV-1 usually occurs only once a year. In addition, the likelihood of there being shedding without an actual outbreak is much less with genital herpes caused by HSV-1. But as you saw in Julie's case, just because herpes usually reacts one way doesn't mean it will always react that way.

Herpes is more prevalent in women than in men (approximately one out of four adult women have it, while only one out of five men do); in men who have sex with other men than in heterosexuals; and in lower socioeconomic populations. The rate is much higher among African-Americans (45 percent) than among whites (17.6 percent). The segment of the population where the growth of herpes is the highest is young, white teenagers.

How You Get It

Genital herpes can be transmitted only by having sex with an infected person. Any fears that people may have about catching it from a toilet seat or wet towel are unfounded. If you ever hear about someone to whom this supposedly happened, you can be sure that the way that person actually caught herpes was by having sex with an infected partner who did not show any symptoms, so that neither one knew that herpes was present. In such cases it might appear as if the herpes was spontaneously generated, or was caused by a visit to some strange bathroom, but that's just not the case. The real cause is that the infected person's skin came into contact with the other person's skin at a time when the infected person was shedding viruses.

Shedding

Let me add few words about the term *shedding,* as I don't want to leave you at all confused on this important concept. As you might expect, if there are visible herpes blisters, then the virus can be transmitted to someone else who comes into contact with those blisters. But it turns out that while those blisters are a clear warning signal, they're not sufficient. Several days before a blister appears, the area in which it is going to appear will be teeming with viruses, which are fully capable of transmitting themselves to another individual. In that scenario, the person is said to be shedding viruses. And in some cases a blister will not arise at all—at least not one big enough to be seen—but the infected person will still be shedding, or giving off viruses, from a particular spot on his or her body. This is called *asymptomatic shedding*. It is more likely that such asymptomatic shedding will be in an area that has mucus, such as the vagina or anus, than on any old patch of skin. And it has been found that some people, in particular some women, shed viruses from their vagina as much as 40 percent of the time, even if they show no visible signs of a herpes outbreak.

The medical community doesn't know exactly how often a person with herpes may be shedding without visible symptoms, but here's one statistic that will give you an idea of the dangers such asymptomatic shedding poses. In one study of "discordant" couples—that is, couples in which one person has herpes and the other doesn't—70 percent of the cases in which the partner without herpes caught the disease were caused by asymptomatic shedding. So while visible indications of shedding can be important indicators, it's those invisible ones that will get you in trouble.

Increased Risk of AIDS

Herpes is not life-threatening the way AIDS is, but it can increase an infected person's chances of getting AIDS. It is no accident that in parts of the world where herpes is endemic, HIV is also widespread. Certainly the sexual behavior of the population has a lot to do with it, but since herpes is more easily communicated than HIV, and then facilitates the transmission of HIV, one cannot discount too greatly the effect that herpes has had on the spread of AIDS. It is also believed that people already infected with herpes who get AIDS have a more difficult time fighting this second virus.

Transmitting Herpes to Newborns

While the biggest danger posed to adults who get infected with HSV is that they become more susceptible to HIV, herpes can also cause very serious consequences to the newborn, and there are approximately 2,000 to 5,000 such cases a year in the United States. However, once again this is a case about which the common belief, even among many doctors, is closer to myth than reality. You may have heard that a woman who has an outbreak of herpes needs to have a C-section when giving birth to protect the baby, as the baby could catch herpes when passing through the birth canal. This can happen, but only in a small percentage of cases because if the mother has acquired genital herpes before the third trimester of pregnancy (twenty-four weeks), then she will pass on to her baby the antibodies that her body has made against herpes, so that the likelihood of the baby getting herpes on its way through the birth canal, even if the mother has active lesions, is very small. (Since it's not impossible, however, a C-section is still recommended.)

The risk to the baby is greater if the mother first becomes infected with the herpes virus during her pregnancy, particularly during the third trimester. Under those circumstances, she will not have built up the antibodies to pass on, and the likelihood of the baby catching herpes, particularly if there are blisters during labor, is much higher, and the potential consequences much more severe than for an adult. It could even potentially cause the death of the infant. For that reason, if an expectant woman has any doubts that any partners with whom she might engage in sexual activities after she is pregnant could have herpes, she should abstain from sex during the later part of pregnancy (third trimester) or insist that a condom be used (while realizing that condoms do not offer complete protection). And since most herpes victims don't know it, I would actually advise that she use condoms with any partner other than one who has been a long-term partner who she is sure is disease-free or one who has been tested with negative results.

By the way, I've spoken to several gynecologists who've told me that time and again pregnant patients with herpes don't tell them about it. Please, if you are in this situation, this is no time to be embarrassed. You must tell your doctor, even if the father of the child does not know. Your doctor will work with you to protect your privacy but for the sake of the baby, it is vital that you tell your doctor that you have herpes, or even suspect that you may have it.

Prevention

I just mentioned condom usage and said that condoms did not provide complete protection. Considering my reputation as an advocate of safer sex, the issue of protection requires a much more detailed explanation.

I'll start with the good news: The HSV-2 virus cannot penetrate a latex condom, so if someone has a sore, or does not have any obvious symptoms but is still shedding viruses on his penis or in her vagina or in either partner's anal cavity, a condom does offer protection. So what's the bad news? The first, and most obvious, is that sometimes condoms break or slip off, and in such instances, their protective value disappears. Using a condom with a viricidal cream on it may give you some added protection if a breakage occurs. (Except to prevent pregnancy, current spermicides are not recommended to be used with condoms, as they may increase the risk of acquiring HIV.) Also obvious are the risks posed by sores that are not in an area that is protected by a condom. Genital herpes sores can be found almost anywhere in the genital region, including the thighs or, as we saw with Julie, buttocks, and so in such instances condoms do not offer any protection. Another is that while latex condoms are impermeable to viruses like HSV, condoms made of lambskin are not. They have tiny holes, too small to allow a sperm to go through, but large enough for viruses to penetrate. And, finally, while a condom will protect a woman if the man has herpes blisters on his penis, it might not always work the other way around, that is to say if the woman has sores inside her vagina. When a woman is aroused, her vagina provides lubrication. That lubrication may contain HSV and if it leaks out of the woman's vagina during intercourse and gets onto the man's genitals or thighs, which are not protected by the condom, then transmission can occur.

Of course, herpes can also be transmitted before intercourse even begins and a condom donned. If the two partners touch each other's genitals as part of foreplay, which is quite likely to happen, then the viruses from an infected person could easily be transmitted to his or her partner. And since a person with herpes can be shedding viruses before any blisters actually appear, there would be no way of knowing ahead of time that this activity was dangerous.

A recent study demonstrated that chronic suppressive therapy with valacyclovir reduced the risk of transmitting HSV-2 to a partner by almost 50 percent. This benefit was above and beyond the reduction of transmission by abstaining during outbreaks and using condoms.

So you see, protecting yourself against herpes is a difficult proposition, which is why so many people have it. The best way to protect yourself is to make sure that any potential sexual partners have been tested, found not to have herpes, and have not had sex with anyone since being tested.

Stephanie—I contracted it unknowingly from a man I loved; someone with whom I *thought* I had a monogamous relationship. Fidelity, it turned out, was not exactly his "best thing"— apparently he got the virus and transmitted it to me without realizing he had it. At least I honestly hope that was the case— I'd really hate to think that he knew.

Suzie—Talk about a hand reaching from the grave. This pretty much confirmed that my ex, father of my children, whom I had suspected, had cheated on me at one point, and gave me "the gift." Certainly he didn't have a clue he had it, or had given it to me.

I went eleven years without a breakout, since the "first time" I had the signs. I then began to break out several months in a row, from January to June, until the doc prescribed a maintenance dose of pills and cream for the next six months (five pills every day for six months straight).

How can you guarantee that your partner hasn't slept with anyone else? You can't, and that's a big problem. You'd certainly never know it if it's the first date because you won't know this other person very well at all, so avoiding one-night stands is a good way of protecting yourself from herpes, as well as from every other sexually transmitted disease. But even if you've been going out for months, as happened to Stephanie, there are still no guarantees. Some people are very convincing liars, and just because they swear up and down that they've been faithful doesn't mean they have.

Another Possible Pitfall

There's another pitfall to protecting yourself against herpes that you might encounter; this has to do with the testing process. When you go to a doctor and ask to be tested for sexually transmitted diseases, the tests may cover many different diseases, most importantly HIV, but the test for herpes is not automatic. You have to specifically ask that you be tested for herpes to make sure that you are. So someone you meet might say to you that they've been tested for STDs and that the results were negative, and yet they still might have herpes and not know it. They'll find out when they get a call from you saying that you've come down with the disease, but that will be too late to protect you. Some of the current herpes serologic tests are not able to distinguish infection with HSV-1 from HSV-2. Because the majority of adults in the United States have a history of cold sores due to HSV-1, a type-specific test (one that can reliably distinguish antibodies for HSV-1 from HSV-2) is important to correctly diagnosis HSV-2 infection. A positive type-specific antibody test for HSV-2 almost always indicates genital infection. HSV-1 antibodies may be present due to oral or genital HSV-1 infection. Serologic tests are unable to determine the site of infection for herpes.

There's another loophole that the herpes virus sometimes uses to get around the testing process. Some of the tests for genital herpes show only whether or not there is HSV-2. So if someone has a case of genital herpes that was caused by HSV-1, he or she may not know they have a genital HSV-1. Therefore if someone tells you they've been tested negatively for genital herpes, ask if they've been tested specifically for both HSV-2 and HSV-1, as well as for other sexually transmitted diseases.

If there are no active lesions, this is not as easy as it sounds. When there are active lesions, a viral culture can be performed and the doctor can determine whether or not herpes is the cause and what type of herpes is involved. You should be aware, however, that how the viral culture is handled is very important, and a false negative is possible if the viruses are somehow destroyed before the test is performed. Overheating of the sample is one such danger. One test, called the PCR DNA test, has a higher overall level of accuracy, so ask your doctor which test he or she is giving you.

If there are no active lesions, then the tests look for antibodies. There are two type-specific serologic tests available: HerpeSelect ELISA and HerpeSelect Immunoblot, both by Focus Technologies. One way the virus might skip detection from these tests is if the infection is too new for sufficient antibodies to have built up. It could take as long as three months after the initial infection for there to be sufficient antibodies in your bloodstream for the tests to be effective.

A more accurate test is called the Western blot, which is 99 percent effective in differentiating between type 1 and type 2. This test requires that the blood be well protected and sent to a lab, and the results may take a while. The cost for this test is also considerably higher than the others. If you think that you might have herpes but the tests your doctor is giving you don't show it, then ask for a Western blot.

The entire testing process is even more complicated than the rough sketch I've drawn here. That's why the most important piece of advice I can give anyone going to be tested for herpes is to find a doctor who is familiar with the process. Having a doctor who performs these tests regularly significantly increases your chances of getting the right diagnosis. So make the effort of getting a referral to a doctor who specializes in herpes; that way you're sure to get the best possible treatment.

Herpes and Couples Trying to Conceive

I've been talking about the importance of condom usage, but what happens if a couple wants to have a baby? Certainly they can't expect much success if they're using condoms. But if only half of the couple has herpes, how can they protect the noninfected partner from catching the disease if they're not using condoms? The answer is for the person with herpes to use valacyclovir, which will offer protection against transmitting the disease, as I mentioned earlier and will get into some more later on in this chapter. This drug doesn't offer 100 percent protection, so there is some risk of transmission. Because of this risk, the couple should be extremely careful. For example, if it is the woman who has herpes and she knows that her menstrual period can trigger an attack, the couple should refrain from having unprotected sex at this time of the month, which is not a fertile time in any case. Being extra careful will probably mean that it will take the couple longer to conceive than if they didn't have this worry, but I think it's worth it in the long run.

While there is no evidence that taking antivirals while trying to conceive would cause any harm to the embryo, such couples should keep careful track of any possible pregnancy. Doctors recommend that pregnant women not take a drug like valacyclovir during their first trimester of pregnancy, so as soon as she knows that she is pregnant, she should stop taking the drug and the couple should rely only on condom use to protect her partner, or abstain from intercourse altogether.

What the Doctor Can Do for You

As I've said, there's no cure for herpes, but just because you have a bad case of herpes doesn't mean that you have to suffer. Although the pharmaceutical companies continue to search for a cure, they've already come up with drugs that will lessen the impact of having the disease. Someone with only a very mild case, one that he or she might not even notice, will probably not seek out such treatments. But if you have a bad case of herpes, there's no reason to suffer needlessly.

Episodic Therapy

There are two ways your doctor and you might decide to treat herpes. The first is called *episodic therapy*. What that means is that at the first signs of an outbreak you tell your doctor, who prescribes a medicine, such as famciclovir, that will reduce the severity of the symptoms. This treatment works by disrupting the process by which the herpes virus reproduces itself and spreads to other cells in the body.

Suppressive Therapy

The other method is called *suppressive therapy*. For this type of treatment you take medicine every day to help suppress outbreaks before they occur. People on suppressive therapy may go for six months or longer between outbreaks. This type of therapy might be appropriate if you have frequent or severe outbreaks, or if herpes has caused you psychological issues, so that you are always very anxious or worried about having a future outbreak. Taking medicine every day offers you the feeling that you are taking control of the situation, rather than allowing herpes to rule your life. This distinction can be very important to some people with herpes, as it allows them to go forward with their life rather than feel trapped by herpes.

Important News

As I indicated earlier, the makers of one drug against herpes, valacyclovir, had anecdotal evidence that people taking it daily were not only having fewer outbreaks themselves, but were also protecting their partners. They conducted a study of almost 1,500 couples, which backed up the anecdotal evidence, and in the fall of 2003, they received FDA approval for doctors to prescribe valacyclovir to reduce transmission as well as relieve symptoms.

This is important news if you're in a "discordant" couple, where only one of you has herpes. In such situations, both partners are going to worry about the transmission of herpes. That's only natural if you care for each other. If you have herpes, you may even worry more about giving it to your partner than he or she is worried about getting it.

And it's equally important if you have herpes and you're not in a couple. Taking any antiviral medication daily doesn't guarantee that you can't give the disease to a sexual partner but the study showed that it reduced the risk by 75 percent, which is significant. The risk is still high enough that you have to tell a potential partner, but being able to tell them at the same time that the risk is relatively small will make a big difference. (All the couples in the study were otherwise healthy, meaning that they did not have any immunosuppressant diseases, and they all used condoms.)

In upcoming chapters I'll be tackling the issue of how to tell a partner that you have herpes, which you'll see has both difficulties and what have to be seen as silver linings.

Chapter Highlights

1. There are two types of herpes, oral and genital, but because of the increase in oral sex, it can be difficult to tell which type you have.
2. Most people who have herpes don't know it because the symptoms are so mild.
3. Genital herpes does not always recur in the same part of the body, which can increase the odds of transmission.
4. Getting tested is not as simple a procedure as it sounds. To ensure that you get correctly diagnosed, be sure to use a doctor who is familiar with the disease and the testing procedures.

2
Coming to Grips

Mark—Getting herpes is like the emotional response after someone near to you passes away. There's shock, loss for something that passed away, a longing for your former lifestyle, a realization that you're no longer invulnerable.

Getting bad news is never easy. And how you'll react to it isn't predictable. You might have a strong negative reaction the instant you receive the news or you might go numb for a while, and then get a delayed reaction that may be more severe than if you'd shown your emotions right away.

The worst reaction you can have is to stifle your emotions because that will lead to other negative effects that you may not even realize are occurring. What some people do after a traumatic event, like the loss of a loved one or a diagnosis of some disease, is to attempt to bury any emotions that they may feel about this event. They do that because they are afraid that they'll go over the edge if they allow themselves to give in to their feelings. They believe that they won't be able to cope with their grief or their fear and so they bottle those emotions up (often with the help of some numbing agent like alcohol or drugs). But since it's difficult to filter out only some emotions, these people cut themselves off from feeling any emotions whatsoever. They'll refuse to even love anyone because of this exaggerated fear. That's why in the long run, rather than try to contain your emotions, it's much better to let them out, and the sooner the better.

On the other end of the spectrum are those people who have an exaggerated reaction, letting their emotions get the better of them and turning molehills into mountains. I don't recommend that path either. You'll scare away just about anyone who might be able to give you emotional support, and then dealing with these overblown emotions by yourself will be doubly difficult.

But a little misinformation can induce anyone to overreact to bad news. For example, the very word "cancer" is quite scary, but some cancers are easily treatable while others can be fatal within a short time. If you react merely to the word "cancer" without listening to the rest of the diagnosis, then there's a good chance that you'll panic, possibly needlessly.

The word "herpes" can have a similar effect, and often does. Many of those who are told that they have herpes by their doctor immediately assume that their love life is over. They jump to the conclusion that no one will ever want to date them because they've contracted this awful disease. To them, it's as if they'd been branded with a bright red *H* on their forehead, and they expect other people to shun them. Here are some examples:

> **Anna**—It has now been almost one year, and I thought I would never again love or be loved. I felt unworthy of love. I felt dirty. I felt damaged and betrayed. At times I was certain in my soul that no one would ever want me. I still have those feelings, but they have lessened in their intensity.

Curtis—When I got herpes I was certain that dating had suddenly gone from difficult to totally impossible. I was sure I was doomed to be alone forever, untouchable, undesirable. It was very traumatic.

Neil—After I realized I was infected, I changed a lot. I felt like a leper.

But while herpes can trigger such thoughts, the truth is, they're not valid. With the right support, both medical and psychological, you can get on with your life, even your love life. As you'll be reading in this book, many people have actually had better success finding a true partner after they've had herpes than before. So why do people feel so bad when they find out they have herpes? First of all there's herpes' reputation. They might not know exactly what that reputation is all about but they know it's bad. Really bad. After all, the media once made a really big deal about herpes. If it was on the cover of *Time*, it must be terrible. So by their reacting to what they believe they know about herpes, rather than the actual facts, their reaction is much worse than it needs to be.

The second problem is that many people who are diagnosed with herpes are not given enough information from their doctor, and far fewer receive any psychological support at all.

Busy Doctors

Let me say a word, at this point, about dealing with doctors. As we've all experienced, the doctor-patient relationship has undergone some major upheavals. With so many people now covered by some sort of HMO, doctors are forced to see many more patients than before, and so there is a tendency to rush you out the door

as soon as possible. That situation is not conducive to the trans-
fer of information.

Viv—Ever since I started to get outbreaks, I would tell my fos-
ter mother and she would take me to the doctor and the doctor would tell me that it was an ingrown hair or that I was allergic
to my soap.

Meigan—I went to a doctor at a different university clinic for a
yearly Pap smear, had what I thought was either the beginnings
of a yeast infection, or maybe a mild herpes outbreak. I mentioned this to the doctor and I was told "You're too nice a girl
to have herpes; a yeast infection will cause this kind of irrita-
tion as well." (I thought that was just a terrible thing to say to
anyone, especially since no tests were run and the doctor could
have been wrong. . . . Then what would that make me, no longer
"a nice girl"?)

Would a doctor give a wrong diagnosis just to keep from hurting a patient's feelings? As these examples show, the answer is yes,
they would. Doctors are not robots. They have feelings and though
they're not supposed to bury their heads in the sand, sometimes they
do in order to "protect" their patients from the truth. And since
herpes isn't life-threatening, there isn't a cure, and testing done too
soon after the initial outbreak won't show up positive in any case,
some doctors may feel that it's better not to look too deeply to see if
it's herpes, because even just hinting that it might be will upset their
patients. These doctors know that if a patient does have herpes, he
or she will get another outbreak and when that person comes back,
the doctor can then run tests.

It's not a good excuse, but it happens because doctors, like all
of us, try to avoid emotional scenes. You can't entirely blame them if
they'd prefer that you do any wailing and moaning outside of their

consultation room. They're not psychologists, after all. What irks me is that in general they don't refer their patients to psychologists when there's a clear need.

In any case, I believe you're better off not getting overly emotional in the doctor's office. If you hear the words "You have herpes," or any other disease, you will become upset, and at that point you won't be able to absorb much of the information the doctor might tell you anyway.

So how should you handle your emotional reaction? I recommend that you compose yourself, go home, and then allow yourself to vent whatever emotions you may be feeling. If you need to cry, then cry. If you want to scream, then scream. But once you've allowed yourself to let off this steam, the first thing you must do is call your doctor and make a new appointment. By the time you see the doctor again, you'll have had a chance to digest this news. If you've been given a prescription, you can get if filled and then read whatever literature comes with it. You might do some research on your own. You should definitely write down a list of questions you want to ask your doctor, so you won't forget anything important. And if need be, you can even bring along a friend or relative, who won't be as emotional as you might be and will have an easier time comprehending what the doctor has to say. Bring paper and pen so that you can take notes, or have the person you bring take notes. And if you have any doubts that you're not getting the best possible treatment because your doctor isn't all that familiar with herpes, or any disease you're diagnosed as having, then find a doctor who is and make an appointment to see that doctor.

Avoiding the Mess

Stephanie—The doctor was telling me that they didn't want to get involved in anything messy like blame, so they declined to tell patients that they could, in fact, narrow the time frame of infection, if they were having a primary outbreak. I was furious, and immediately found a new gyn.

Stephanie offers another example of how some doctors do their best to stay out of their patients' personal lives. Appropriate testing can help the patient find out who gave them herpes, but that could then lead to a major blowup, and there are doctors who don't want to get caught in the middle, particularly if there could be any legal implications. They're wrong to shirk their responsibilities to avoid complications, but you have to be aware that it does happen.

Misinformed Doctors

Betsy—There is so much misinformation out there. Most doctors don't seem to understand enough to teach their patients.

Betsy's comment is one that was given to me again and again. So while some doctors shoo their patients out the door because they don't have the time, and others because they don't want to deal with an emotional scene, there are also some doctors who do it because they just don't know enough about herpes. I can't tell you how widespread this is, but it really is inexcusable. Any doctor who is unsure of himself or herself should refer their patient to another doctor who does have the necessary expertise.

Alan—The lack of support and the ignorance in the medical community is one of my pet peeves. I've heard over and over again from people with herpes that their doctor told them that the Western blot test is only for AIDS, when in fact it's the best test there is for herpes. Since I'm in marketing, I've taken it upon myself to try and do something about it. I've written to doctors and used my own money to get the word out to the local medical community about the various tests and treatments for herpes. I know other groups have done the same.

The wonderful thing about our society is that there are so many people who volunteer their time, effort, and money to get things done. Because of my European background, I have the tendency to trust authority figures like doctors. But there's nothing wrong with the can-do spirit enjoyed by Americans and I applaud those who've taken the time to volunteer with the many support groups and get the word out to both laypeople and doctors.

And whether or not you ever become a group leader, at the very least you should follow their examples with regard to your own medical needs. Yes, the doctor-patient relationship has changed, but that doesn't mean that you can't figure out a way to get effective treatment within this new system. The difference is that you can't expect to lay all of the responsibility on your doctor. You have to shoulder more of the burden, but I think that when you do that, you'll feel yourself more in control of your illness (and this advice goes for any illness, not just herpes), and this will actually aid your recovery.

Your Emotional Response

As you work with your doctor, you'll be able to find the right balance of medical help to alleviate the physical symptoms of herpes. But where does that leave you with regard to the state of your emotional health? Over time, herpes attacks lessen in intensity, but the damage done to your psyche can be much worse if left untreated.

Anna—No matter what people tell me about how it's no big deal and not everything is herpes, it is a big deal.

Many people do get depressed when they learn they have herpes. And the more they dwell on such thoughts, the deeper their depression becomes. It becomes one of those vicious cycles so that their herpes colors everything they do in a shade of gray.

> **Amanda**—Because I knew there was no cure, I was sure that I'd never be able to meet anyone again. My life was doomed. I decided it wasn't worth it. I wrote a suicide note. It was the day of the O.J. verdict. I went to NYU because I'd taken some classes at the film school and I remembered they had nice big windows. I went up to the eleventh floor, found an empty classroom, opened a window, and sat on the ledge for over an hour. Then some people came into the room and I left and went to my therapist's office.

There are some whose spirits descend so low that they consider suicide, and some people actually do commit suicide every year because of a diagnosis of herpes. The latter may already have been severely depressed, and the diagnosis of herpes merely served to send them over the edge, but the depressed states that many herpes sufferers fall into were not there prior to their diagnosis. It's a direct response to having caught this virus.

Other Emotions

> **Mark**—Half the people who get herpes want to commit suicide and the other half want to commit homicide.

Depression isn't the only emotion that herpes can trigger. Many people feel tremendous amounts of anger well up inside of them. Anger directed at the person who gave them the disease; perhaps at every member of the opposite sex; at the medical community for not having a cure; and in some cases even at the world at large. Anger can not only make it difficult to stabilize your emotional well-being, but it can even cause physical ailments such as high blood pressure.

Sometimes anger can be as hard to deal with as depression. Because herpes keeps coming back, it can trigger bouts of anger each time, and they could even get worse. If that happens, don't hesitate to get some counseling for it. It's not something that should be ignored, particularly because it does take a toll on your body.

> **Viv**—It's been so long that I have allowed myself to be attractive to someone that I don't know what is right anymore. Because of my shame and guilt, I don't want to go there.

Another emotional response to herpes is a feeling of shame. Before you got herpes, you probably thought that the only people who got this disease were low-lifes; "normal" people like you would never get something like herpes. And that shame then attacks your self-esteem, because if you have herpes, what kind of person does that make you?

You might also feel guilty. Guilty for what? Guilt is a strange emotion because it can arise when there's absolutely no reason. Someone stands directly behind you with a cup of coffee and you turn around and bump into them, causing the coffee to spill all over the other person, and what do you feel? Guilt. But was the accident your fault? No, not at all. So you may feel guilt about having herpes, even though you did nothing wrong. You're the victim, and yet you feel guilty.

> **Anna**—I thought my life was over when my doctor told me I had herpes. I isolated myself from people, and tried to maintain a sense of normalcy in my daily routine and with work. I

looked at people around me and wondered who else had it. I saw a ten-year-old girl with a cold sore and thought, "She has herpes, and she'll have to tell someone someday."

The likelihood is that your emotions will actually swing back and forth. First you may be depressed, then you'll get angry, and when the adrenaline of your anger wears off, you'll be depressed again. You'll be walking down the street and feel guilty and ashamed, even though no one around you is even aware of you, much less thinking about what a bad person you are for having herpes.

This roller-coaster ride of emotions makes it harder to recover your sense of well-being. Where you might be able to handle one emotion, having your emotions gang up on you this way makes you feel more and more out of control. And restoring the control you had before herpes struck is what you want most.

The best way of coping with these emotions is to try to put what has happened to you in its proper perspective. So the question you have to answer as calmly as possible is where, on the scale of bad things that may befall you, does a diagnosis of herpes actually fall? I don't want to minimize what's happened to you, but I hope that by the time you've finished reading this book you will no longer be looking at this diagnosis as signifying the end of the world.

Of course, each individual's reaction will depend on a variety of factors, including his or her psychological makeup, personality, and background. But exactly how those factors will combine when mixed with a diagnosis of herpes cannot be assumed with any certainty. For example, one might logically conclude that a very shy person who gets herpes from the first person he or she has ever had sex with is going to have a harder time dealing with this disease than someone who is very outgoing and gregarious and has dated lots of people. I agree that in general that would be true, so that someone who is bright and bubbly all the time would have learned over the years how to put aside negative feelings and accentuate the positive. But there will also be cases where the opposite occurs. Outgoing people may feel as if they have more to lose. If someone has never had a problem getting a date, he or she may be more psychologically dependent on having a social calendar that is filled to the brim. The shy person, on the other hand, who ends up withdrawing deeper into his or her shell will actually be retreating into a place which is familiar and even "homey." Such a person might even feel some relief, saying to himself or herself, "I never much liked the dating scene and now I have a good excuse not to force myself into doing something that made me uncomfortable." In the long run they certainly won't want to spend their entire lives alone, but for the time being, they might not feel so bad about having gotten herpes.

Compare that to outgoing people with a brand-new case of herpes who, after spending just one weekend alone at home, will feel as if they'd been tossed into solitary confinement in a cramped, dank dungeon with a lifetime sentence. Thinking such thoughts will make them even more morose and they could find themselves on a slippery slope that could lead to a severe case of depression.

I'm not saying that this must occur, only that it might. My basic point is that you can't be certain how you'll respond to different stimuli. But the other side of this coin is that no matter how you actually respond, there are also ways of countering the negative aspects of getting herpes. All you need is someone to show you the way, and I trust that this book will help light the path.

There Is No Cure

Mary—I was in the doctor's office and he walked out and there was a chart on the wall that listed all of the sexually transmitted diseases. I walked over to it and looked at what was written for herpes and saw that there was no cure. I thought, "Oh my God," and then I started crying hysterically.

One of the big psychological pitfalls of herpes, maybe even the biggest one, is that there is no cure. You may have heard of people who have gotten other sexually transmitted diseases, like syphilis or gonorrhea, but assuming those people took care of themselves and went to the doctor and took all their medications, then they were probably able to successfully rid themselves of whatever it is they caught. That won't happen to you, at least not until medical science comes up with a breakthrough. Once you have herpes you have it for life. But remember, there's HAVE and there's have.

If you read Chapter One, then you know that herpes outbreaks tend to get less and less severe over time. So while the herpes virus may still be in your body, your body will develop antibodies that will have some success in doing battle against the disease.

Betsy—I think daily suppressive therapy should be offered to everyone from the moment they are diagnosed. It really helps you to cope with it if you aren't having painful OBs interfering with your life. The fact that it helps to protect your partner is just another great reason to take it, in my book.

But no matter how strong those antibodies of yours may be, they don't have to fight by themselves. There are medications that can be quite effective. If you can afford to take them every day, then you may never have any further attacks once the medicine has gained control, or when you do have them, they'll be very mild. But even if you take medication only when you have an outbreak, or when you think you're going to have one (more on that later), then you'll still have a great deal of control.

Curtis—I started taking oral antivirals every day. Because they gave me a feeling of control. I didn't have to constantly worry about having an outbreak. I hadn't wanted to have it so badly that I needed to take pills every day for the rest of my life. This was a big issue for me. But between my doctor and my support group, I got up the confidence to try it and it really turned things around for me. Suddenly I was able to break this cycle where every time I thought about my sexuality I would think about herpes. And then when I got married, it was wonderful not having to worry so much about giving it to my wife.

These medications do more than just keep the symptoms of herpes from driving you crazy. From the psychological point of view, their most important strength lies in their ability to keep safe any partners you may have who do not have herpes. Even with these medications there is no 100 percent guarantee that you won't give a partner the disease, but the odds can be significantly reduced, and then, if you also take every precaution, they can be reduced even further.

Prodome

Amy—Many people feel genital itching before they get an outbreak, sort of like an allergic reaction. Others have a burning in their thighs or flulike symptoms. My feet itch before I'm going to get an outbreak.

As I've already mentioned, using condoms is one important way of not transmitting the disease. But as I also pointed out, condoms do not offer complete protection, especially as an outbreak can occur on places like the thighs or buttocks that are not covered by the condom. But what many victims of herpes have discovered is an ability to predict when an outbreak is likely to occur. They can sense that the herpes virus has become active even before there are any visible signs. The feelings that they get are known as *prodome*. Either taking medication or abstaining from sexual contact during those times has proven to be an effective protective mechanism.

Predicting an Attack

Even before the effects of prodome can be felt, it may be possible to predict an oncoming herpes outbreak. The key is to carefully observe your body in order to determine what factors might trigger an attack. By keeping a diary, you may be able to trace some patterns in your life that seem to always precede an attack. For example, while the medical community has not proven that stress leads to outbreaks, most people who have herpes will tell you that it does. So if you have a fight with your boss and the next day you break out with lesions (or several days later, if that's how your body reacts), then that would be evidence that stress did cause you to have an outbreak.

By the way, stress can take many forms. It doesn't always have to be emotional. I was speaking with a personal trainer who told me that she had a client who would have a herpes outbreak if she worked out too strenuously. So for this woman, putting stress on her body physically is a trigger. I've also heard that certain foods can trigger a herpes attack. Too much sunshine is another possible trigger. And many women report that having their period, which can cause all sorts of different stresses, triggers attacks. Since there is a wide variety of potential triggers, only you can find out which of them might apply to you, which is why taking note of your daily activities is an important component of taking control of this disease.

Dealing with Anger

Gayla—Every time I had an outbreak, the hatred would stir up in me, especially for my ex-husband for giving it to me. And the physical pain stirs up even more emotional pain. When it hurts to simply go to the bathroom, I get so angry with him that I curse his name. Because herpes isn't life-threatening, some people think it's not so serious. What they don't realize is that it steals your life from you. I can deal with the physical pain. What I can't stand is feeling like a leper.

Some patients who come to me and hear me tell them not to be angry about something or other tell me, "But Dr. Ruth, I can't help feeling angry." To a very small degree, I agree with that statement, but definitely not entirely; let me explain why. If something triggers an angry thought about someone else, say following a new outbreak of herpes, then it's true there is nothing you can do about that initial burst of anger. In the heat of the moment, you're going to feel angry. But please note the word "moment." You have my permission to be angry for a minute or two with the person who gave you herpes. I'll even give you dispensation to say a curse. But then you have to push that anger out of your mind. How? By filling your brain with some pleasant thoughts.

What thoughts? It's hard for me to tell you what thoughts would work best for you as I haven't lived in your shoes, but my telling you what I do may give you some ideas. I keep a drawer filled with things that give me pleasant memories. Pictures of my children when they were young. Mementos from vacations. Ticket stubs from Broadway shows I particularly enjoyed. So when I'm angry, or sad, or frustrated, I open that drawer, pull something out, and contemplate the pleasing memories that object evokes. Then I go on with the rest of the day in a pleasant mood instead of with a scowl on my face.

Whether you need some actual objects to push those unpleasant thoughts aside or can do it just by focusing on something inside your brain is up to you. It will take a certain amount of effort and concentration, but once the nasty thoughts are fading, you'll see that it's fairly simple to keep them away.

What's a Behavioral Therapist?

In order to get you to believe me at this point, let me tell you a bit about what I, as a behavioral therapist, do to make those people who see me feel better about themselves. First of all, I still see clients in my office. So if I give advice, it's not stale. That's important to me because there have been changes in our society and old advice might no longer work. And, by the way, among my clients have been those who came to me because they were suffering from the psychological effects of herpes, and I've been able to help them.

My job as a behavioral therapist is not to change people but to change their behavior. I don't psychoanalyze them. I don't probe their minds. I do ask them very personal questions, especially when doing sex therapy, because it is vital for me to find out what the problem is. Then I give my clients homework, actual things to do, that can improve their quality of life. I know that these methods of modifying their behavior work because they come back and report what happened. So when I tell you that you can deflect your anger, please believe me.

Of course, it's possible that you won't be able to do this by yourself. You may need some additional support to get you over this hump. One important way of getting this support is by joining a herpes support group. I'm going to tell you a lot more about that in another chapter. But while there are many support groups, they're not in every city. And even if there is one that is near to you, you still might not be able to attend their meetings. For example, some people work nights, and these meetings are usually held in the evening. Or you might have children and can't afford a babysitter. Or you are taking care of an elderly parent who can't be left alone. The problem with group meetings is that the time of the meeting is set to accommodate the largest number of people, but that's not going to work for everyone. But finding a therapist who can meet you at an hour that is most convenient to you is a lot easier. Therapists cost more money than support groups, which charge only nominal amounts, but behavioral therapy isn't exorbitant, particularly because it is short-term, and it's well worth the cost if it can bring you some peace of mind.

So in order to get a grip on your herpes, you have to first get a grip on yourself. You have to figure out the best way of taking back as much control over your life as possible. As you learn to control your emotional response to this disease, you'll find that you'll be better able to adjust to the physical aspects of having herpes. You may not be able to cure yourself, but you can promote so much healing that instead of herpes being like a giant weight tied around your neck, it will be more like a light chain with a small charm attached to it.

Chapter Highlights

1. Herpes isn't a death sentence. Accepting that you can have a fulfilling life even with herpes is the most important step toward healing yourself psychologically.
2. Take charge of your treatment. Not only will this help you from a medical standpoint, but it will also help you psychologically.
3. You can control your emotions. Learning how is an important step in coping with this disease.

3
You Are Not Alone

I told you in Chapter One that there are an estimated 60 million people in the United States with genital herpes; six million of them know that they have it because they've noticed outbreaks, ranging from mild to severe in nature, and the rest don't. But since herpes is not something that people brag about, or in many cases even whisper about to their best friends, having all those people out there who are sharing your misery is not of much comfort if you don't know who they are and can't communicate or commiserate with them. But what if you could? Wouldn't that be great?

The fact is that you can. Not with all six million of them, but with enough that you'll feel a lot better with your situation. There are sixty support groups sponsored by the American Social Health Association. You can look up one near you on their Web page, *www.ashastd.org*, and for those of you who don't have access to a computer, I've printed the list in Appendix A of this book. As you might imagine, these groups are concentrated in major cities, so if you live far from one, it might be difficult for you to attend regularly. But if you are having difficulties coping with herpes, then if you can go to even one meeting, I would suggest that you make the attempt. I'm going to pass on some of the stories of people who've gone to these meetings, and I know it will be helpful reading them, but they can't match up to the real thing.

What's the main asset you'll gain by attending such a meeting? If you're feeling guilty and ashamed at having caught this disease, then seeing what the other victims of herpes look like, and then hearing them talk about their experiences, will lead you to the obvious conclusion that these are perfectly average individuals. And if they're quite normal, then that will help you to accept that you're quite normal as well, and that having a case of genital herpes doesn't make you a bad person who should go around hanging your head in shame.

The reason that I know this visit will be helpful to you is because that's what happens to most of the other herpes sufferers who've attended one of these meetings. They go in filled with trepidation and they come out with new confidence. One meeting might not be enough to bring them all the way back to their former selves, but it can form the foundation of their psychological recuperative process, which is why I'm advising you to make every effort to attend at least one such meeting. And, of course, if you find that you get a lot out of that one meeting, you'll put in the extra effort to go to some more.

Now I don't want you to listen only to me on this subject. I've spoken to many people who've gone through this process, and here's what some of them had to say:

Ann—After I discovered that I had herpes I turned to my friends for support, but since they'd never had it, they weren't much help. The first time I went to a support group I was petrified. I didn't know what I'd find behind that door. I was expecting a bunch of freaks. I was so relieved when I saw they were down-to-earth people. I learned so much from the group, about medications, what foods not to eat, all sorts of topics. I made some really good friends and learned to accept myself and my circumstances.

Ann's is a fairly typical case. She found it hard to get information about herpes and she was "petrified" about going to a group meeting. The fact is, you will have to push yourself to overcome the psychological barriers that herpes erects but if you do, you'll definitely find it rewarding.

Curtis—Going to a support group gave me perspective. I didn't have any friends who had it, so I thought my situation was unique. When I discovered how many people had it, I was staggered. After that I stopped feeling so alone, so unique. I also was taught what questions to ask my doctor. When I'd left his office the first time all I had was a tube of some sort and a gaping hole filled with questions. After that first meeting, I was able to focus in on what was important to ask my doctor.

Your doctor should be a partner in helping you deal with herpes, but as I pointed out, doctors are being forced to devote less and less time to each patient. You have to really maximize each second you have with your doctor and to do that you have to come armed with a base of information and questions. By hearing about other people's experiences, Curtis was able to focus on getting the answers he needed.

Anna—I somehow found my way to a local help group. I was terrified to enter that room. As I walked in and gave the door person my name for a name tag, I thought I would choke on my own breath. I didn't want anyone to know my name. Then it occurred to me that they were all here for the same reason. It was one of the hardest things I have ever done.

Time and again people reported that going to their first meeting was the most difficult thing they'd ever done. That's not surprising, as there are two separate fears operating. The first is personal. By entering, you're admitting to whomever is there that you have herpes. If you've been keeping that fact a secret, then this will be hard for you to do.

> **A.T.**—People come with preconceived notion that they're bad or dirty. What we try to convey to those folks is that they have contracted this virus by doing nothing more than what 99 percent of the population does, engage in sexual activity.

The other fear is that of the unknown. What will these people be like? Even though you now have herpes, some of the prejudices about people with herpes will affect the way you think about other people with herpes. So until you cross that threshold, you're probably going to have some negative feelings about this group of people with herpes. You're going to imagine that they're creepy in some way, even if you know better. So walking through that door is not going to be easy.

> **Neil**—It took me over a year to go to my first support meeting. I was still carrying around a lot of hurt, confusion, and some anger from not having talked about it much. I had a really bad time that first night because I'd been stewing about it for over a year so I went home and prayed and asked God to show me how to make it right. The next night I decided to go back and make as many women in that place feel attractive and desirable and alive again as I could. I succeeded on a limited level, though some people just don't want to hear it.

You'll be learning more about Neil in later chapters, but he's someone who got on with his life after herpes, talking to friends about it and managing to date women and talk about it, but it wasn't enough to overcome the emotional damage that herpes had done to him. He needed the help of the group experience to further purge himself of the psychological pain he was carrying around.

> **Amy**—After I found out I had herpes, I was a wreck. There was an eight-hour period when I thought I'd take my own life. I was so upset, I couldn't even type the word "herpes" on a keyboard. A girlfriend did some research for me and found that there was going to be a large meeting right in Indianapolis called the Indy Gathering. I was scared to death of going but my friends talked me into it. One even stayed at my house so that there would be someone there for me when I got back. (She was so great, she even cleaned my house while she was waiting.) When I walked into that room I thought, "These people are far too happy to have herpes. This must be a cooking class." People tell me that I was one of the angriest people ever to walk into one of their meetings. Craig, one of the founders of the Indy Gathering, came up to me and said: "How are you?" and my answer was "I hate anything with a penis." He said, "Okay, we'll work on that." He now uses that as an example. That was on a Friday night. By Sunday I was crying as I was saying good-bye to these people who literally had saved my life.

Amy could have gone off the deep end because of herpes. All her emotions became supercharged. She has supportive friends, as you can see, but because they hadn't gone through what it's like having herpes, they really couldn't supply her with the counseling she needed. Luckily for her she was able to attend a large group meeting soon after she contracted the disease. And even more luckily, she met Neil there, and they're now a couple.

While each person who attends one of these support group meet-ings will be bringing a different set of problems, anyone who goes can find enough information to get significant help. Also, although most people go to a few meetings, get the help they need, and then stop attending, the group leaders are committed individuals who have heard all the stories and can be extra helpful in getting an individual over some of the tougher humps. They provide an invaluable resource that you couldn't find anywhere else. As you saw in the case of Amy's group leader, Craig, he wasn't upset at hearing Amy's reaction to him as a man, but instead was able not only to help her overcome her bit-terness toward the opposite sex, but also to file her case away to be used to help other people. So if you go to a group, you can be certain that no matter what your reaction is, the group leader has likely dealt with others who have had similar reactions. He or she will have the experience to help guide you toward a solution.

Anonymity

By the way, even I was not allowed to attend a meeting in my area. These are very private discussion groups limited to people with herpes. So don't worry about revealing that you have herpes to the world just because you attended one of these meetings. The only people who will know you've been there are people who also have herpes, and in many support groups, you can remain completely anonymous, so that no one has to know your real name. So don't let the fear of letting the word out stand in your way.

The Importance of Experience

I'm someone who believes experience is very important in treating people. When a client comes to see me with a problem that I feel

I'm not experienced enough to handle, I always refer them to someone else. Yes, I've been a therapist for twenty-five years, but if I've
never handled a particular problem, I can't possibly do as good a
job as someone who has treated dozens, if not hundreds, of people
with a similar case.

To me, finding the right person to refer them to is the most
important thing I can do for them. It's why I also believe that if
someone has a medical problem, he or she needs to find a doctor
who has handled many such cases successfully, because that doctor's
experience is more valuable than any training. You need book learning to get started, but there are skills experience can teach you that
are impossible to learn from a book.

What experience brings to someone in the helping profession
is feedback. If I give someone advice about a particular sexual problem and they come back to me and say it worked well, or it didn't
work, then I can use that information when addressing others with
the same needs. My clients aren't guinea pigs to whom I'm giving
advice hoping that it will work, but rather part of a long series of
people for whom the behavioral assignments I give them have
proven themselves time and time again. When a therapist is just
starting out, he or she has to rely on the experience of others that
has been handed down through books and lectures, but as someone whose very first client was a handicapped young man—for
which my training had been on the light side, shall we say—I can
personally testify that there's no substitute for experience.

Your Friends

Ron—After all of these years, and during the divorce process, I
decided it was time for me to *effectively* deal with H. I decided
to talk with others about the emotions, fears, rejection, and
social stigma associated with H. Talking to select friends about

H was a relief. I finally found the acceptance of others who did not have H. Some actually had H and had never revealed it to anyone, and others knew of others who had it. Even though many of my friends were supportive, they couldn't really understand what I was going through unless they had H themselves.

On the other end of the spectrum are your friends. As you saw in some of the cases I've presented, friends can be very supportive, especially in Amy's example, where they played a valuable role in getting her help. But as Ron points out above, if they're not experienced with herpes, they can help but they cannot *really* help you solve the emotional upheaval you are going through. And to a great degree, this advice applies to almost any situation you might face. If you have a parenting problem and you ask a friend who's a parent for advice, they will only have parented one set of children, their own. They are experienced, but perhaps not experienced with your particular difficulty. If their children are doing well in school and yours aren't, for instance, any advice they may offer could be wrong for your child. In some cases that won't be true. If you ask a parent of a child who's already had a teacher that your child is having difficulty with, they might be able to provide you with significant insight. So I recognize the assistance that friends can give and I'm not telling you to definitely refrain from asking your friends for advice, only encouraging you to go for professional counseling if the problem persists.

And despite being a therapist who gets paid for rendering service, I don't consider professional advice to come only from a paid counselor. Herpes support group leaders are certainly well qualified, as they have a lot of experience with herpes. Religious leaders may have helped lots of couples get through a rough spot in their marriage, for example. A social worker at a hospital might have saved many battered women from further abuse. So while I encourage you to get help any time you face some psychological crisis, if need be, I would also encourage you to dig a little deeper into the pool of potential caregivers in order to find a qualified person you can afford.

Jane—I talked about having herpes with many of my friends. Then, when I was starting to date a doctor whom another of my friends was interested in, she went and told him that I had herpes before I got the chance to. So from that experience I've decided that it's safer not to tell anyone you're not sleeping with that you have it, unless you're in an anonymous support group. It's not a good idea because people who don't have it may not understand.

I don't believe that Jane's example is typical, but it could happen and so it's something you have to consider. You do need to talk about your problems with having herpes, and a support group is a fairly safe environment in which to do that, particularly if you remain anonymous. But hopefully you also have friends you can trust. Of course, if they start telling other people, then the news may travel like wildfire, and if that news infects your local dating pool, that can be a problem. As you'll learn later in this book, if you do a good job of telling a potential partner about herpes, the odds are that person won't run the other way. But if they hear about your condition from someone else, particularly someone who doesn't have your best interests at heart, then their reaction to you is probably not going to be a positive one. So be careful whom you tell, and make sure that you say to everyone you talk to that what you are revealing is confidential. That's not a guarantee that the news will remain private, but if you don't say that, the friends you do reveal this information to might not be able to guess that you want it kept private.

Meigan—Eventually having to date again brought about a more open, sharing view, especially when I tried to explain to some of my girlfriends why I still had not had intercourse with a certain boyfriend yet. Explaining living with herpes was a lot easier now that I knew for certain that is what I had, and I educated myself about it so I could talk intelligently about it.

Eventually you are going to begin feeling more comfortable about telling people that you have herpes. You may never want to walk around the streets with a sandwich board advertising that fact, but there might come a time when you find keeping the secret more of a burden than revealing it. This will depend on your personality. If you're someone who could never resist telling your friends the least little details about your life, then you're going to have a hard time shutting them out of a huge chunk of your life after you get herpes. But someone who has always protected their privacy may decide that there is never going to be a time when they're going to let their friends know that they have herpes, and that's okay too.

> **Betsy**—I've found that my friends knowing I have herpes has been a great way of dealing with it for me. When I have an OB I can be honest with my friends instead of lying, which is a great stress relief. Recently one of my friends came to me and told me that even though she knows I have herpes too she only just now could tell me she and her husband have it too. She's been so embarrassed to have it that she's never told a soul besides her doctor and her spouse. She says it's been really helpful to talk to me about it and she's learned more about herpes since she told me than she had in all the years she's had it. It's being able to help someone I care about like that that allows me to be open about having herpes. A secret can only hurt you if it is a secret, in my book.

As Betsy says, talking about a problem is a good way of relieving stress, but while I do urge you to talk about it, because of support groups, and online chat groups, it doesn't have to be with the people you are friendly with or work with. It is possible to relieve yourself of some of the psychological burdens of having this disease while also maintaining your privacy. You have to do whatever feels comfortable to you.

Leaning on Your Family

While family members can be of great help, they also pose a risk. If you were to go to a friend and tell them you have herpes and they reacted badly, then that friendship might come to an end. Of course that would be sad, but as you went on with your life, this incident would fade in its importance. Family members, on the other hand, are with you for life. Even if there's someone you decide you never want to speak to again, that will still pose problems, over and over. Holidays, weddings, and other family gatherings can become awkward, and family feuds end up spoiling everyone's enjoyment.

> **Ron**—Telling a family member was very hard. After literally watching a cousin die of AIDS, I heard all of the jokes that my family members told. I can remember the laughter, blame, and the insincere sympathy that they displayed toward him. After watching all of that, I just knew I couldn't tell any of my family. It wasn't until ten years later that I decided to tell my sister. I was crying, and I just told her. After revealing everything inside, she told me that me having H didn't even matter because she still loves me because I'm her big brother. That really meant a lot to my self-esteem, knowing that I had someone who loved me for me regardless of what's inside my body.

In Ron's case, even ten years after he'd been dealing with herpes, it was difficult for him to tell another family member. Why?

Because if his sister had had a negative reaction, he might have damaged one of the most important relationships he had. To Ron, it was bad enough that he had herpes, but if this disease had caused a rift between him and his sister, it would have been that much worse.

Rebecca—When I was first diagnosed at twenty-two (three years ago), I didn't know who to tell, who to turn to, or where to turn to. I turned to my sister, who is twenty years older than I and also one of my closest friends. She supported me. She told me she'd find online groups that I could refer to and some educational websites. I've told my mother, and some of my friends, and the reaction I get from them are questions! Never anything negative, just questions.

I'm not telling you to never go to a family member for help with a problem. For many types of problems, such as financial issues, they may be your only source of assistance. But when dealing with something about which you feel embarrassed, like herpes, I suggest you consider carefully before unburdening yourself to a family member. If you are close to a parent, grandparent, sibling, or aunt or uncle, a relative who has always given you helpful advice and support through the years and whom you can count on to be discreet—the type of relationship that Rebecca had with her sister—then by all means go right ahead and talk to that person. Just remember that if he or she doesn't know that much about herpes, that person may not provide a very deep font of the right knowledge to tap into. But if that relative can give you some much-needed comfort, as well as maintain your privacy, then don't hesitate to open up the lines of communication. Someone close to you like that brings the added value of real love, for which there is no substitute when it comes to comforting someone who is hurting. But if you're considering talking to a family member whom you haven't approached for advice before, then lay out the pros and cons before you go to that person. If there's even a 50/50 chance that the final outcome will make you feel worse than better, then keep your mouth shut. That's especially true if a negative reaction will then spread quickly among your entire family.

Maybe there will come a time when you'll want to let your family know that you fell into the same trap that herpes has laid for so many millions of others, but you might want to wait until you've gained some emotional control over the situation before having to deal with having to face a family full of questions. You also want to make certain that you have all the facts down. If you still have a lot of questions, how are you going to answer the questions of your family members? But if you've already learned a lot about this disease, and can answer their questions with confidence, that will definitely affect the way they think of you after they learn this news.

Herpes and Your Place of Employment

When I was writing this book, I thought that perhaps there would be important issues regarding herpes and people's place of employment. I suspected that there might be repercussions, depending on whether word got out or the secret remained hidden. For example, if you changed jobs and the new insurance company asked you about existing conditions, what effect would having herpes have? I was sure people would be reporting problems in this area. But in asking around—and some of the group leaders sent out e-mails to large groups—nobody reported having any such problems.

This was not a scientific survey and I would strongly advise that you check your own place of employment. You don't have to tell anyone that you have herpes. Just check to see if there are any ramifications whether you tell or not. Certainly if you are getting reimbursed for drugs to control your herpes, that is going to be on some record somewhere. But since herpes isn't a disease that will lead to expensive hospital visits, perhaps it is of no real consequence when it comes to such insurance issues.

As to telling any friends you have at work, I would advise some caution. If you don't want the word to get out, make sure that you only tell people who are discreet. Your fellow employees are in some ways similar to family. As long as you have that job, you will be seeing them regularly. If someone decides to be nasty about it, there's not much you can do. So in a case like this, it's better to be safe than sorry.

Chapter Highlights

1. While it may seem that you are alone, there are people to whom you can turn for help.
2. Support groups offer expert advice and anonymity.
3. Be careful when discussing herpes with family, friends, and fellow workers. Being discreet may pay off in the long run.

4

Silver Linings

Suzie—I'd rather have herpes and be alone than be in a relationship with a stupid person.

Herpes builds character.

Herpes is an internal radar system for being more selective and for making better choices in weeding out jerks who aren't worthy of my time and friendship.

There is no cure for stupidity.

Stupidity is deadly.

Herpes isn't.

When the first few people that I interviewed mentioned the "silver lining" of having herpes, I was rather skeptical. Getting herpes certainly shouldn't be looked at as desirable, and I was afraid that if I started talking about this silver lining, people wouldn't take this book seriously. As I've said, I don't believe in scare tactics, but I also don't believe in coddling people. Having herpes is not pleasant, and if potential readers thought I was going to sugarcoat this experience, especially if they'd already had a rough time of it, then they'd want nothing to do with my book on the subject. And I wouldn't blame them, either. But then, as more and more people repeated the same thing, I had to take this silver-lining concept more seriously.

Let me begin by saying that this silver lining isn't so wonderful that it would make someone go out and catch herpes on purpose. Also, it's not just one thing, but a series of different benefits, not all of which any one person may end up using. But taken together this silver lining can be quite valuable, especially if you know to look for the various ingredients that can be a part of it and figure out how best to use them. That's why against my first instincts, I'm devoting an entire chapter to this subject, because I would not like for you, assuming you have herpes, to miss seeing this potential for making something positive out of what certainly starts out being quite a negative.

Old-Fashioned and a Square

I'm proud to admit that I'm old-fashioned and a square. This attitude comes in part from being brought up in an orthodox Jewish home as a child and spending most of my early years in Europe and Israel. It also comes from being 75, a status that I'm proud to have reached, though I wouldn't mind being a bit younger. (In Hebrew we read from left to right, so I feel that I can tell people that I'm really only 57 without seeming too dishonest.) These two ingredients of my personality, my background and my age, mean that while I'm aware of what's happening on the dating scene from what I read and what people tell me in my private practice, I'm not entirely comfortable with it. I know intellectually that many individuals are having sex without first forming a relationship, maybe even without knowing the other party's name, but I can't bring myself to condone such behavior. There are too many negative ramifications, like the spread of STDs, which I believe are a mistake to ignore. That's why I continue to tell anyone who will listen that people should form a relationship before they have sex. But I also know that many people aren't paying heed to that message.

One of the reasons I'm against casual sex is that it isn't really casual. More often than not, at least one half of the coupling couple has some feelings for the other. And if that phone doesn't ring within a few days of that sexual episode, the person with those feelings is going to feel bad. Perhaps they shouldn't have gotten sexually involved so quickly, but peer pressure can act like a steamroller and be very hard to avoid. Many people who decide to have sex after only a date or two hope that having sex before a relationship has fully developed will make it more likely that it eventually will, though that rarely happens. And conversely they are afraid of losing a potential long-term partner by saying no to sex. That does happen, but I don't think the odds of a short romance developing into the love of your life are so great that they make up for the negative aspects of casual sex.

The bottom line is that many people are having sex in a matter of days or weeks, instead of months and years. There are many in this group who think this is a good thing. These are mostly men who have no desire to commit and plenty of desire to have a variety of sexual partners. This is a situation built for them, especially if they're willing to use some sweet talk to cover their real intentions, which are only to have sex. But there are also women out there who share this view of sex as a sport. They've learned how to have orgasms, they enjoy this "power," and so they use it. I believe that in the long run both sexes are going to regret this type of behavior, but there's not much I can do to prevent this from taking place besides advising against it.

If these people looking only for sex paired off strictly with others with the same view, then the negative effects would be mitigated. The problem is that they often prey on those looking for relationships, and it is the ones in this second group who end up getting hurt. And, of course, sometimes they also wind up with an STD. So what do these changes in the dating practices of young people, and some older ones too, have to do with the silver lining I mentioned that comes attached to getting herpes? Potentially a lot, because herpes can act as a brake that may counteract, to some degree, this disconnect between sex and relationships.

> **Shannon**—My best piece of advice came from the nurse in the ER, who said something along the lines of, "I have a friend who has had herpes for many years and she sees it as a blessing. It weeds out the good guys from the bad guys. If they are a good guy, they like her for who she is and the herpes doesn't matter. If they aren't, then they aren't worth her time anyway." I thought about that for a while, and it seemed strange to count herpes as a blessing! But the more I thought about what that nurse said to me, the more I realized it was very true. So I adopted that philosophy for my own life and went on. I decided I had a long life ahead of me yet and I wouldn't let getting herpes stand in my way. I also realized that I couldn't live with *not* telling somebody if I was interested in a relationship and/or sexual involvement with them. I would be putting them into the same situation that my ex-boyfriend had put me into when I was seventeen.

So by having to have The Talk, Shannon must force herself to take a much closer look at any potential partners. And that applies to anyone with herpes. So while it's still possible for someone with herpes to have a one-night stand, having an STD does raise the bar with regard to such couplings, because you still have to tell this other person that you have herpes, at least if you have any sort of a moral compass. Of course, if you're both drunk or high that won't make much of a difference, but under normal conditions, herpes will be a sobering thought for some and so should slow the process down.

And since I brought up the subject of morals, getting herpes certainly can be a kick in the butt when it comes to reappraising your own morals. How can you be mad at the person who gave you herpes if you then don't tell everyone that you are putting in danger of getting this disease? I know that there are some people who still don't tell, maybe even because they're so angry that they see giving it to others as a type of revenge, but in such cases, their anger has grown to a point where it is more closely akin to a mental disease and has pushed aside much of their personality. But for most people, I believe their true self will eventually emerge and they'll do the right thing when it comes to telling others about the risks.

Curtis—After getting herpes I had something that forced me to make myself very vulnerable beforehand. It raised the bar on the relationships I could have. Now, suddenly, I had to be able to have an intimate conversation with someone before there could be any physical intimacy. I wound up getting to know people first, so the quality of the relationships improved, as did my success at finding somebody for a long-term relationship.

It would be great if we all had the willpower to always do what is right, but let's face it, most people give in and take the easy way out at least now and then. For example, some people don't lose the extra weight they've put on until they develop a disease like diabetes that makes that extra weight life-threatening. Or they don't learn how to handle their finances until they're forced into bankruptcy. It's part of human nature. People who are having sex without a long-term relationship know that they shouldn't be behaving this way, but since the possibility is there, they give in. And it's particularly difficult when the process of finding a long-term partner involves going through short-term relationships. More often than not, your next date won't become your next long-term partner. But even though this person might not be appropriate for a long-lasting relationship, it's easy to drift into having a short-term sexual relationship. But, again, herpes can be the force to change you so that you develop the back-bone to say no and put the necessary effort into finding a true part-ner. And the end result is that you'll be better off for it. And even if all it does is extend the time period between when you first meet to when you first have sex, that's still a positive. The longer you know someone, the better you'll know them, and so even a slight exten-sion of time could prevent you from making a big mistake.

> **Mia**—One thing I must keep telling myself: "It's not HIV or AIDS." I will live and I will have a fulfilling life. I was in a horri-fying situation, but it was also a wake-up call. I wouldn't de-scribe myself as promiscuous, but I didn't really have standards when it came to satisfying my physical needs. I figured, "I have everything I need for me at this point; what do I need to be in a serious relationship for?" I was no longer in a long-term rela-tionship, so I didn't have to sacrifice or do for anyone other than myself. I took care of business and had lots of fun.

Mia points out another part of this silver lining. She took chances and got herpes, but it could have been AIDS. So getting herpes can be used as a wake-up call to yourself so that you re-move this risk from your lifestyle. To my way of thinking, that's a very important part of this silver lining. There was a time a few years ago when AIDS was keeping people from risky behav-ior, but then along came some of the miracle drugs, and people started getting careless. First of all, those drugs can cost as much as $30,000 a year, and while insurance can help, that's not al-ways the case. Furthermore, there are now strains of HIV that are becoming resistant to these drugs. So having a casual attitude about getting AIDS is becoming as big a mistake now as it was back in the '80s. And while in the '80s AIDS was a disease that affected almost no one but homosexuals, now it's become so widespread that anyone is at risk.

There's another aspect to this issue. I know it can be hard to ask a potential sex partner about the state of his or her health. Asking someone if they have an STD implies something negative in their character, even if you know that's not true because you got herpes without being a promiscuous person. The person you ask might get insulted anyway, and then you'd risk losing this person. And it's especially hard to bring up the matter of testing for STDs if some passion has evolved. If this potential partner has never been tested, by the time he or she makes an appointment and gets back the results, weeks may go by. If you're both getting very hot for each other, those weeks may seem like an eternity. And if the other person ends up taking a pass, then it *will* be an eternity. But if you have herpes, then you have a perfectly good excuse to bring up this subject in order to protect this potential partner's health. And after you've revealed that you have herpes, there's a natural transition to asking about the other person's health.

Even though you have herpes and have to have this talk, you'll still have to stop and take a deep breath before you begin to have this particular conversation. If you end up having to have this sort of conversation many times, it will get easier as you get more experienced, but you'll never be completely relaxed since you can't know ahead of time how this person will react. Rejection is always a possibility, and since being rejected is always painful, it's quite likely that you'll flinch before revealing that you have herpes.

And whether or not the other person decides that furthering a relationship with someone who has herpes is possible or not, they're going to be at least somewhat shocked by what they hear. Certainly no one is going to jump up and down when they hear this news, unless, of course, they have herpes, or some other STD, and they were equally worried about having to tell you.

So at least for a few moments, there is going to be some awkwardness after you make your revelation. But if you've handled this tactfully and in such a way as to cause the least amount of negative thoughts in the other person, and if you're prepared to wait for the other person's reaction, then this sort of experience won't be the worst in the world for you. And if having such a conversation ends up saving your life because it prevents you from getting AIDS someday, then that's quite a silver lining when you think about it.

> **Gayla**—The feedback that I get from having The Talk has been a great benefit. First of all, most people will compliment me for my honesty and that's a good feeling. But their reaction also allows me to see all sorts of things about them. I can tell if the person is educated or uneducated, if they are open-minded, willing to learn, compassionate. All sorts of qualities become apparent that otherwise it might take me weeks or months to find out about.

As I said, most people are going to be a bit shocked when you make your announcement. That means their reaction won't be totally under their control. You know how you watch every word that comes out of your mouth when you're first dating someone. Everybody does that. You know that first impressions count and so you hide behind a mask for a certain time. But when someone hears something surprising, that person may not be under full control, so you're likely to get a more honest view of them. If, as Gayla said, their reaction is one that leaves you less than enthralled, then you'll know that this person would not make a good long-term partner and that you're better off not wasting your time with them.

An Aside

The following has nothing to do with herpes per se, but it's part of my philosophy and I want to pass it on. First of all, the most precious gift we have is time because we only get a fixed amount in our lives, and there is no way to tell in advance how much it will actually be. So in my opinion, time is not an asset that you should waste.

One major way that people waste time is on dead-end relationships. Think about some of the relationships of people you know that were doomed, almost from the start. Think about your own past relationships and how many of them were mistakes. To me, if a relationship is not going to lead to something substantial, then it's not worth continuing. Since I'm old-fashioned and a square, to me "substantial" means *marriage,* but that doesn't always have to be the case. But it should at least be a relationship that could lead to marriage. Anything less is a waste of your precious time. Rather than be in a relationship that is going nowhere, you should get out of it and find one that will be more substantial.

As I said, this applies to anyone. Of course, it's not always easy to tell where a relationship might be headed, especially in the beginning. But part of the herpes silver lining is that you may find out sooner rather than later, as we've seen. But it does you no good to say to yourself, "This person is not right for me," but then continue to see them. I know that perhaps because you have herpes you feel that you should be less selective. If someone is willing to continue the relationship, no matter how lousy a relationship it is, it's better than nothing. Well, I respectfully disagree. If you're not going to be happy, and if it's going to end at some point anyway, then don't get involved to begin with.

Anna—On the other hand, it's a gift to be able to accept yourself and know you can move on and grow from it. My goal is to grow as much as possible from this. I do not have cancer, AIDS, or any other life-threatening illness. I have a happy life otherwise; I have worked through many of my problems successfully. I have good days and bad days, and I know I can't change what has happened. The one resolve I do have is that I will not let herpes control my future. I am still scared and apprehensive, but willing to move forward.

My boyfriend said he thought he had arrived earlier for me than I did for him. Meaning, he knows he is worthy of love and I have not yet fully realized that. But he knows it, and reminds me of myself daily. If I had to receive the "gift" of H in order to arrive at the moment of meeting him, then it really is a positive gift. Without intending to sound clichéd, it makes me appreciate even more what is left of my life and what I have today. My mantra is that I have H. Sure, it stands for Herpes, but it also stands for Hope.

Anna is living proof of what I'm saying. She recognizes how little time we all have and she's making the most of it. Yet there are many people who waste their lives not just in staying in dead-end relationships, but also in looking down on themselves and not trying to make the most of those precious hours they have on earth. So if it takes getting herpes to make you appreciate your life, then that, too, is a silver lining.

Thinking Positive

It's easy to concentrate on the negative. Often it's the negative parts of your life that force themselves on you. If you have an outbreak of herpes, you're uncomfortable, at the least, and perhaps even in pain. It's not something you can ignore. So when herpes lesions are making themselves felt, it would be very easy to feel negative. I recognize that you can't stop negative feelings from occurring. In the case of a herpes outbreak it's perfectly legitimate to feel downright lousy about it. But I'll give you this permission for only a limited amount of time. That's right, after a few moments of feeling sorry for yourself for having herpes, or whatever nasty thing has just happened, you have to pick yourself up and start thinking positive thoughts.

Not easy to do, you say. Perhaps, but I say it's not impossible either. And once you get the hang of it, it becomes easier and easier. Don't think I'm taking your suffering lightly, because I'm not. I lost my entire family in the Holocaust and I almost lost both my feet during a bomb blast in Palestine, so I understand pain. But I also know that you can't give in to pain, whether it is psychological or physical. You have to acknowledge it, but then you have to find a way to move beyond it.

On one of my television shows, I had as a guest a man who's a quadriplegic. Do you know what he talked about? How great his sex life was. Certainly he has a very hard life, and even having sex with his wife is not easy, but he does have sex and he does enjoy it. He wasn't going on TV to complain about being a quadriplegic but to show all my viewers that almost anything is possible if you have the right attitude. So that's what I want you to develop, a positive attitude. Despite herpes, or maybe because of herpes. It doesn't matter the reason behind it, just that you do it.

"Dr. Ruth," I hear some of you saying, "how do I develop this positive attitude, especially when I'm in pain?" That's a legitimate question and it wouldn't be fair of me to simply tell you to do something and then not tell you how. I could simply send you back to Chapter Two, where I offered advice on how to avoid being angry, because what I said there does apply here. You have to push those negative thoughts out of your brain with some positive ones, and I told you about the drawer of mementos I keep for a "rainy day" when I'm feeling sad. But I've got more up my sleeve than merely that drawer, so here are some other ideas. Some may seem obvious, but if you've never used them to lift your spirits, then I guess they're not as obvious as they seem.

Play some upbeat, happy music. Sad songs make you cry, as we all know, especially if we're already feeling sad, and happy, uplifting music can make your spirits revive. If you get into a blue funk regularly, I might suggest you create your own CD or tape that contains nothing but upbeat songs. That way you can be sure that for the next sixty minutes or so, your brain will be getting nudged in the right direction.

And it can also help if you dance to the music. In fact, any type of exercise can lift your spirits. Your body creates endorphins, which are mood elevators, when you exercise, so even though you may be tempted to crawl under the covers, get out and dance or run or jump and you'll quickly start to feel better.

Just as music can set the mood, so can lighting. A great mood enhancer is to go out into the sunshine. The problem with that is that there may not be any sunshine when you most need it, either because of clouds or because it's nighttime. When that happens, you have to rely on artificial light. If your home is not well lit, then go out and buy some lamps, and maybe add some dimmers, so you can change the mood as you see fit. You might even make one room especially bright for those days, or nights, when you really need a lift. I've read those ads for lamps that supposedly give off the same type of light as the sun and that are supposed to be mood enhancers. I don't know if they work, but they might be worth a try.

Another quick fix, for at least some people, is to put some flowers around the house. Their bright, vibrant colors can help lift your spirits. You can either get one large arrangement and sit near it, or else buy several smaller ones that you can put in various rooms. If you're the type who can get a positive vibe from the right smell, then be extra choosy and pick flowers that will give off an aroma that you find pleasing.

Some friends tend to bring you down when you speak to them, while others instinctively know how to lift your spirits; I would recommend calling one of the latter, if you can't actually get together. You can tell this person that you're feeling down, but then don't keep the conversation on that subject, but instead talk about other things—past times that were really funny, for example—that will put you in a better mood.

Some people seek comfort in food, alcohol, or drugs, but those are just illusions. You may be able to elevate your spirits, or at least forget your troubles, for a short time, but eventually those troubles will come back even stronger. If you don't naturally head in one of those directions when you're upset, don't start now. And if you have a problem with one of these substances, then seek professional help.

Finally, there's my specialty, sex. Indulging in a great sexual fantasy can do a lot for your mood. During the time you're fantasizing, your other problems disappear, and while they may return afterward, they won't be as strong and will be more easily pushed aside. But sex, like food, alcohol, and drugs, can be abused. There are people, most of them unhappy people, who spend hours every day masturbating. That's not a good thing to do. Eventually the sexual stimulation you get from masturbation starts to lessen and then it's of no use. And to waste hours a day doing anything, even something as pleasant as a sexual act, does not suit my philosophy. What about sex with a partner? I'm all for that, but remember, your partner is not necessarily sharing in your mood, either the part of you that is upset or the part that is seeking sex. If a partner turns you down, that may make you even more upset. So be careful if you turn to your partner for solace through sex. Don't approach them as if it was a given that they'll say yes, but rather hold some of your emotional commitment back so that you don't sink even further if sex is just not something that they are ready for at that time. But I am sure that your partner will give you a hug any time you need it, and hugs can make you feel a lot better too.

Amy—After I got herpes, someone told me this story. He thought that oysters were born with a pearl inside of them. Then he found out that wasn't true. They have a hard shell and a soft fleshy inside. It isn't until some irritant, like a grain of sand, gets inside that shell that they grow a pearl. Oysters have nerve endings and the grain of sand causes them discomfort, even pain, very much like getting an STD. The oyster deals with this irritant by secreting a liquid, layer upon layer, that hardens, and the end result is a beautiful pearl. So the process produces something of great beauty and value. That's what herpes has been for me. I almost took my own life at first. Then, by adding layers and layers of education about herpes, I was able to turn it into something of great value to me.

Amy says that you can take the fact that you have herpes, a negative, and slowly turn it into a positive by learning as much as you can about it and making changes in your life accordingly. The key word here is "slowly." The oyster doesn't make a pearl overnight. I don't know how long it takes, but on the scale of an oyster's life, I'm sure it's at least years. So while there may be a silver lining in your life from having gotten herpes, don't expect to find it right away. It may take you some time to heal, both physically and emotionally. It will definitely take you some effort, either by learning facts or just by learning about yourself. In other words, you have to develop this silver lining and not just expect it to drop into your lap. That's excellent advice with regard to almost everything you do. Just look at the whole process of education. It takes years and a lot of hard work to get a degree, but then you have something of real value. So it's definitely worthwhile to stop looking with only a negative viewpoint on the fact that you have herpes, and to immediately start searching for any silver linings you might be able to develop from this particular phase of your life.

Ron—Conclusively, living with herpes has been a blessing. I know that sounds strange, but this virus has allowed me to love myself unconditionally. (If I don't, who will?) I just want to say that living with herpes is what you make it, be it a positive or negative. I choose to be positive and make a difference.

Ron has a very positive view, and that's great. He's really been able to look at how his life has changed and he sees nothing but good from that. But as a group leader he also actively went out of his way to do the most good he could do (as have the others who responded who are group leaders). He truly turned his grain of sand into a pearl, and in some sense it was easy to do. Since there are so many people who have herpes, with hundreds of new ones getting it every day, there's a never-ending source of people who need help, some even desperately. They won't reject your help, but instead are like drowning people looking for someone to throw them a lifeline. So for anyone who has had trouble meeting people, joining a herpes group, and taking an active part once you've received the help you need, is a great way to make some major, positive changes in your life.

And most important of all is that it is up to you to find those silver linings. As we've seen, there are people who've gotten herpes and who committed suicide or went into hiding for their entire lives. Those are the worst-case scenarios, but plenty of other people continue with their day-to-day existence but remain miserable, if not forever, at least for years.

The oyster makes a pearl instinctively. Humans have to make a conscious decision to act. We're constantly faced with choices, and some of them are quite hard. There may be what appears to be an easy way out, like locking yourself away from the dating scene because you have herpes, but in the long run, this path of least resistance will lead you down a very difficult road. So if you have herpes, or any other burden, try as hard as you can to find the silver lining and in the long run you'll be able to overcome this difficulty rather than succumb to it.

Chapter Highlights

1. Herpes forces you to have The Talk, which in turn means that you will learn a lot about a potential partner sooner rather than later.
2. Being forced to be open about having herpes could protect you from getting something worse, such as AIDS.
3. It's up to you to find the silver lining that herpes can bring.

5
The Talk

A lthough this is a book about herpes, when it comes to having
The Talk, the same advice applies to all those with any one of
the many sexually transmitted diseases that plague our world. Yes,
there are aspects of herpes that aren't shared by other diseases, such
as the fact that there is no cure and condoms aren't sufficient protection to prevent its transmission, but what most people find difficult
is not the exact words to say—though they are important—but getting any words to come out of their mouth at all. In fact, many people
with an STD avoid dating for a period, which can go from weeks to
months to years to the rest of their life, just because they can't get up
the courage to have The Talk.

A great deal of the resistance people have in revealing to a potential partner that they have an STD is the fear of rejection, which
is natural enough. But also natural, and usually more powerful, is
the urge to find a partner and have sex. So however long the waiting period, more often than not, the majority of people with an STD
end up returning to the dating scene.

Keeping Mum

Some people get around the difficulty of having The Talk by simply not having it. They date, have sex with other people, putting them at risk for catching the STD they have, and usually end up infecting at least some of them. As you no doubt know, even using safer sex techniques, such as always using condoms, won't necessarily protect a partner, particularly when it comes to herpes, as other parts of your body besides the genitalia may also shed viruses. And since condoms can break or fall off, they do not offer 100 percent protection against the transmission of any STD (or preventing an unintended pregnancy, for that matter). It's not that the people who keep their STD a secret don't know that it's wrong, but they all make up some excuse or other for maintaining their silence.

> **Betsy—**I contracted genital herpes when I was eighteen years old. It was one of those college things where I chose a total stranger to have sex with one night. I continued on as usual sexually. At that time HIV was still a gay disease so I didn't even use condoms regularly. One night a friend who I had had drunken sex with told me he had just been to the doctors that week and was diagnosed with genital herpes and it was most likely me he had gotten it from. I was so embarrassed!! By that point I was already involved with someone else and couldn't find a way to tell him about it. I of course was in denial over the fact that I could have any STD, let alone herpes. Unfortunately the guy I was dating contracted herpes from me. We broke up soon after his diagnosis. After that happened I knew I had to tell partners that I had herpes.

> **Jane—**I'm fifty-three years old and have been dealing with herpes for twenty-one years. I'd always been a heavy drinker. My drinking and drug taking got worse. My herpes did too. The

only knowledge we had then was if you didn't have an outbreak, you couldn't give it to anyone. So, my decision was, if I sleep with someone, I'll wait until I see if the relationship might get serious and then I'll tell them. As long as I was careful, I wouldn't give it to anyone. Of course, how careful can anyone be when drunk?

Ron—While in college, I never told anyone. At that young age, I was afraid, alone, and felt that no one would understand. My college years were a time of denial and fear of disclosing. It was like I didn't have H. I even used excuses while I was in relationships, such as "as long as I use protection, then they (women) don't have a right to know." Regretfully, I put others at risk, to appease my own desire and denial of actually coping with H.

Cecelia—I got herpes when I was young and basically ignored the symptoms. I thought they were a yeast infection or something. Then I got married and several years later ended up being diagnosed as having herpes. I was devastated. I didn't know how I was going to tell my husband, David, especially as I was sure that I must have transmitted the disease to him. Luckily for me, he was very understanding, and we ended up taking part in a study about transmission and I guess we didn't get the placebo because David never caught it.

Larry—Would I tell everyone I was remotely interested in sex with that I had herpes? Would I stay celibate until I had met the "right one" and told him all about it, and had been accepted? I felt that not revealing it in any circumstance would be deeply unethical and thus agonized for months. I slowly came to a kind of uneasy moral compromise. If I wanted to play with the rough-and-ready guys who go to sex clubs I would, and would not feel the need to tell, but anyone I met and began a dating or communicative friendship with would need to know if I felt we might be heading toward intimacy. So I had some rough-and-ready casual sex, and also dated a few men, none of whom were fazed by me telling them I had herpes. Indeed a couple of guys I dated replied rather nonchalantly, "Oh, that. I had it once but it never came back."

The majority of the people I've been in contact with do tell potential partners that they have herpes, and most of the time they are not rejected because of it, but I'm not sure that I have a representative sample of people with herpes. In one sense I know that I don't because 90 percent of those with herpes don't know they have it, so how could they tell anyone of the risk ahead of time? But even among those who do know they have the disease, I doubt that the group I contacted represents a clear cross-section. After all, anyone who is not able to deal with herpes to the extent that they don't tell potential partners is not very likely to have volunteered to tell me their story about herpes. That's true even though I guaranteed complete anonymity. So my sampling is clearly skewed toward people who normally do tell, which means I can't give you any percentages or even rough guesses as to how many don't.

Now, since most of you who are reading this book already have herpes, you might think that whether or not people tell doesn't matter to you. But as I said at the beginning of this chapter, these communication problems are not limited only to those who have herpes. There are undoubtedly plenty of people with STDs that you don't have who also aren't telling. And unlike herpes, people with HIV can pass on a disease that is deadly (and it's been shown that people with herpes are more likely to contract AIDS when exposed to HIV than those who don't). So the dangers are plentiful, which is why, whatever you do, make certain that any potential partners can show you the results of having been tested. Remember, even if you show them how honest you are by letting them know that you have herpes, it does not necessarily mean the person you're interested in having sex with will reciprocate. If this person has been lying about his or her health for years, the psychological barriers may be too high for them to get over just because this person has met someone with higher standards.

Looking Back

I've jumped the gun here a bit because before you start telling any future partners that you have herpes, you may also have to tell any past partners. The necessity of doing that will depend on who gave it to you and how many sexual partners you have had since then. Even if you haven't had sex with anyone else besides the person who gave it to you, you still must speak with that person. Why? you might ask. Because there's a good chance that they don't know they have it.

> **Frank**—I had sex with this girl a couple of times and then she called me and accused me of giving her herpes. I told her that was impossible, as I didn't have herpes. But then I thought about it. A few years earlier, I'd had one little pimple on my penis. It went away and I never thought about it again, but then I realized that it must have been herpes. And so it turns out I probably did give it to her.

When I say that 90 percent of people with herpes don't know they have it, that doesn't mean that that they never had any symptoms. Most of them did, but the symptoms were mild and went away by themselves so that a doctor never saw them, and so people in this group never connected the symptoms they had to herpes. It's certainly easy for a woman to have a lesion or two on the inside of her vagina and never know it, as most women aren't looking up there with a flashlight very often. And since yeast infections are fairly common, any itching or other discomfort she could feel she might very well attribute to such an infection. And telling the difference between a mild case of herpes and jock itch or a yeast infection is difficult for a doctor, no less a layperson, to diagnose. So that explains why there are tens of millions of people running around with herpes who don't know it. But just because they had a very mild first case of it, and no subsequent outbreaks, this has no bearing on what will happen to someone to whom they give the disease. That next person may get a very bad case with painful lesions, and he or she is going to be extremely upset at having been given herpes without being told of the risk ahead of time.

So, even though talking to past partners about your case of herpes may not be a pleasant task, it's one that must be done in order to protect the future partners of anyone who might have given you herpes and doesn't know that they have it.

Your Attitude Is Important

Tanya—The advice that I give to those who ask, when it comes to disclosure, is to be calm and honest. Find out all you can about herpes, before you even consider telling any potential partner that you have it, so that you can answer any questions that come up. If you are not comfortable with this, you cannot expect anyone else to be comfortable with it, either.

While this particular form of The Talk is different from the one where you're speaking to a potential future partner, it does share one very important quality, which is that you must be very well informed about herpes, or any STD that you might have, when having this type of discussion.

It's impossible to say how the other person will react. In this particular case, they may already know that they have herpes. Or they might not. Or they might be in denial. Whether or not they know, they might try to lie about it. If you're well informed, you'll be able to build an airtight case so that they will have to, or at least should, admit the truth.

If they don't have a clue that they have herpes, they may react very badly to getting this news. They may be as shocked as you were when you found out, or even more so. Again, being able to answer their questions will make you both feel a lot better, which is why having this knowledge will provide an important boost to your level of confidence. If you can rattle off all the correct statistics and symptoms and facts, then you'll know that you'll be able to respond properly to whatever questions this person may raise. But, on the other hand, if you expect to be saying "er" and "um" a lot, then that will shake your level of confidence and make you even more unwilling to have this version of The Talk.

Of course, bringing along some pamphlets or material you pull from the Web will be helpful tools, but in the end it's the words that come out of your mouth that will be most important, so try to make sure that you really understand as much about herpes, or any other STD that may be involved, as you can.

A Note of Caution

Amy—I got herpes from one of two guys. One was sort of creepy, and while I think he gave it to me, he denied it. The other was a cute cop that I met in New Orleans. I guess I'll never know who really gave it to me, but I prefer to think it was the cute cop instead of the creep.

Unless you've only had one partner in your life, it can be very difficult to know for certain who gave you herpes. Remember, you might have had a very mild outbreak yourself at one point and not noticed it, and that could lead to a more severe outbreak later on. So even if you're absolutely certain that X, your last partner, gave you the disease, unless X was your very first partner ever, you have to admit in the back of your mind that it's possible that X isn't the culprit.

If you believe in your heart that X gave you herpes, it's going to be very tempting to get angry with this person while you are having this talk, but instead you must tread carefully. An angry reaction will not make it easier to get them to admit that they have it, or to get them to go for tests, and so the end result could be that this person will go on infecting others. So I would advise that you make a serious effort to withhold your anger, at least until you get your message across and this person finds out for sure that he or she has or doesn't have herpes.

Those You May Have Infected

If you have had several sexual partners since you were infected, then it's possible that you unwittingly infected some of them, and so you have the responsibility to tell them, both so that they can get tested and treated if they have herpes, and to keep them from spreading the disease even further.

> **Rebecca**—When I first found out . . . I was dating this guy. . . . I had a hard time debating how to tell him, but I cared so much that I did. It scared him off and he was very angry and upset and ended our relationship.

I wish I could tell you that everyone you tell is going to be sympathetic to your plight and won't get upset at you, but I'm afraid that there are no such guarantees. Certainly there are people who'll forgive you and will still remain a sexual partner. Others might not want to have sex again but will remain friends.

But it's also possible that someone will get very angry, even if it wasn't your fault because you didn't know you had it. And even if you think you know this person (which you should, at least to some extent, if you've had sex with them) you can't predict how they are going to react to this piece of news.

Their next step is going to be to get tested, and then you'll find out whether or not you've infected them. If the answer is yes, that may be another opportunity for outrage, though if someone hasn't exploded on first hearing the possibility, it's likely that they'll hold their temper if a diagnosis of herpes is confirmed.

The Legal Implications

In this litigious society of ours, a question that often arises is "Can I sue someone for giving me herpes?" or the converse, "Can I be sued for having given someone herpes?"

I can't give you any definitive answer because ultimately it depends on which state you live in and the laws that apply there, but I can tell you this much: The odds of there being a legal remedy are fairly slim. Most lawyers are not going to accept such a case on a contingency basis, meaning that they won't take on a case like this for a percentage of the final settlement but will want to be paid at an hourly basis for the work they do because they know the odds of obtaining a large settlement are not good. So when looking at $10,000 or more in legal fees, most people who cry "I'll sue" end up not doing so. And since most insurance policies won't cover the losses of such a lawsuit, unless the person being sued has deep pockets, there won't be much money for the victim to get even if they did pay the fees and ended up winning such a suit. There have been some cases reported in the papers that had to do with celebrities who were sued for passing on herpes, which were settled out of court. But unless someone famous gave you herpes, or unless you're famous, the odds of ever going to a courtroom because of herpes are not very great.

Discarding Your Anger

I actually think this lack of a legal recourse is a good thing. I know it doesn't seem fair that someone could give you a disease like this and that there's no legal remedy for righting this wrong, but let me explain my thinking on this to you. Any time you go to court, you can be sure that the outcome won't be decided for years. That means any anger you have for the person who gave you herpes will fester for all that time. Yes, you might get some limited revenge in the end, but the cost to you won't be only in the dollars you spent on lawyers' fees. This fight will also eat at you on the inside. That is going to do you a lot more harm than whatever positive effect the feelings of revenge you may get some time down the road will provide to you. So my recommendation would be to forgo any ideas you might have about suing.

Taking this piece of advice one step further, I would also add that you should stop being angry with this person as soon as you can. Let's say that you believe the person who gave you herpes is lying to you. This person might have said that he or she didn't know they had herpes, even though they knew full well that they did. Let's say that you suspect that's the case. Of course you'll be absolutely furious with them at first, and you could easily allow that anger to bubble along for years. You could get so angry that you go as far as hiring a private detective to find out if he or she had ever given herpes to anyone else so that you could confront this person with the proof of their lie. And even if you didn't go that far, you could toss and turn in your bed at night going over various scenarios of revenge.

You could, but what would that get you? During the time that your anger ruled your life, you probably wouldn't go out and find a new partner, one who would accept you, herpes and all. You'd have plenty of lonely nights to give in to your anger, but would those come anywhere near the satisfaction of spending those nights in someone else's arms? In my opinion, the best option would be to forget about this person, and the sooner the better. In the long run, such bitterness will do you a lot more harm than it will ever do to the other person, especially as there's a good chance that the stress caused by your anger will actually exacerbate your herpes. I'm not necessarily saying you should forgive that person. I'm not saying you shouldn't either, but I understand that might be asking for too much. All I'm suggesting is that you forget this person, and more importantly, the anger that you have for him or her. The sooner you can do that, the sooner the healing process will begin.

The Future

Now that we've dealt with the past, it's on to the future; your dating future, that is. As we've seen, many people who get herpes initially feel that their days of dating are over and that they'll never find their true love. But while that can be the case, it certainly doesn't have to be. Herpes may make this quest harder (and some will even debate that, as you saw in the chapter on the silver lining) but by itself this disease won't keep you from meeting people. The only person who can do that is you. I'm going to go into the ways of meeting people more deeply in another chapter, but since I know that having The Talk is one of the big barriers, I need to convince you that it is not as high a barrier as you might think.

> Jane—I also dated someone who I decided to tell because we had begun to have feelings for each other. I was really nervous telling him. I laughed when I told him, because if I didn't laugh I would cry. He got very quiet. Then I could see, he was very very

angry. I started to tell him I was really careful and that I was sure he couldn't have gotten it from me. Then I started crying. He turned to me and said, "I have it too." He wasn't planning on telling me. The reason he got angry was because in his last experience, he had dated a girl who told him she had it before she slept with him. After she told him, he confessed he had it too. It turns out, she had baited him to get him to be honest, and walked out on him. She didn't really have it and had devised a way to find out if her potential partners did. He thought I was doing the same thing because I had laughed when I said it.

So here I say that it might not be as hard as you think and I start out by giving you a horror story. I chose this example for several reasons. The first is that it's probably impossible to guess what is actually going to happen when you have The Talk. In this case, Jane couldn't possibly have known his history, and she was just laughing out of nervousness, something not in her control.

If you're going to give a speech at work, it certainly makes sense to rehearse it over and over so that you're in control while you're speaking. But in a conversation, once you've thrown out the opening line, where it heads is anybody's guess. There are so many possible permutations that you would get dizzy trying to figure it out ahead of time, and you'd undoubtedly be wrong no matter how much time you spent. So, yes, you have to be prepared with the facts, but don't think that you can actually map out what is going to take place.

The other reason that I chose to put this example first is because this scenario pretty much shows you the worst that you can expect. It's certainly not a pleasant occurrence, but it's not so terrible and it's also avoidable.

Jane—The dilemma now is always do I wait until I'm emotionally involved with someone to tell them, then if it's a big issue and they walk away, which is a choice I respect, I end up hurt.

That has happened to me. Or do I tell them up front before we know each other that well to spare my own broken heart if it is an issue with them. I've done both.

As you can see with Jane, despite having gone through this pretty bad rejection, she doesn't automatically tell people right away to make certain she won't get hurt again. Sometimes she does, and sometimes she doesn't. That shows that the pain, while bad at the time, was something from which she was able to recover. And if she really wants to avoid the possibility of a painful rejection, she just has to have The Talk sooner rather than later in the relationship.

Sex Can Be Easier Than Talking

Curtis—It's often easier to sleep with people than to talk with them.

Curtis is absolutely correct, but when you stop to think about it, how strange this seems. Two people are more willing to take their clothes off in front of each other and touch each other very intimately and have an orgasm in front of the other person than to talk about something like herpes. You talk to people all day long and yet you keep your clothes on in front of them and you don't touch them, beyond perhaps shaking their hands. So why is having this talk so difficult?

Betsy—I was still embarrassed when men knew I had my period at that age so telling someone I had herpes was not easy for me.

Embarrassment is certainly one reason. Even if you know how common herpes is and that you don't have to be someone who sleeps around with everyone you meet to get it, it doesn't mean this other person knows it, or will believe you when you tell him or her.

And then there's the issue of lust. When you're having sex with someone, lust sort of takes over your brain and you may do lots of things that you later can't believe you did. But when you have The Talk, any hints of lust will probably disappear. You're faced with the cold, hard, naked truth, and that can be difficult to take.

The Delayed Reaction

Martha—Usually they'd be great, but then they had to go digest it, and do their own research. The waiting period was always tough. Thought they'd say that you're disgusting, but never got rejected. Always felt tremendous amount of responsibility, burden, paid attention all the time, every little twitch.

Neil—I met a nice young woman who happened to be a nurse. One night I tried to have The Talk, and I was initially rejected. She went back and evidently looked up more about herpes, got informed, and the next time I saw her she was far less rejecting.

It's natural when giving someone a piece of news that you want their reaction to be immediate. If he or she is going to reject you because of herpes, you want to know that right away, or if the relationship is going to proceed, you want that to happen quickly also. As these two examples show, such expectations may not be met.

If you think about it, that makes perfectly good sense. If someone gave you such news, you probably would want to go back home and mull it over in private so as not to overreact. Yes, knowing that you may have to wait to get the final outcome for days, or even longer, will make it a bit more nerve-wracking. But if you expect that wait, just the way you know you have to wait for the results of a blood test after a visit to the doctor, then the initial lack of reaction won't be as bad. On the other hand, if you're anxiously waiting for a final answer and you don't get one, you might feel even worse than if you got a negative reaction. So adjust your expectations to include the fact that you might not get the answer you seek right away.

Neil is someone who says that he had talked about STDs with his partners for many years before he got herpes, so he didn't go into having The Talk without experience. But that didn't necessarily help him when it came to telling people that he had herpes.

Neil—The first time I talked about it with a lady, it didn't go very well for me. Because of the stress I was feeling, I'm not even sure what happened. I didn't really pursue if after that first time so I don't know if she rejected me or whether the relationship never developed because I backed off.

Neil provides us with another valuable lesson here. Remember in Chapter One when I was going over your initial reaction to hearing about herpes from the doctor and mentioned how you probably weren't in the proper state of mind to really hear what he or she was saying? As you can see with Neil, the very same thing can happen when you talk to a potential partner about herpes. If you're very nervous, you might not be able to pick up on the other person's reaction. You might not be able to tell whether it's positive or negative. You might just say to yourself, "Whew, I'm glad that's over with!" and not even care what the results turn out to be. That's typical of the reaction that many young males feel the first time they ask a girl out on a date. They're so fearful of rejection that if they get a yes, they might not even hear it.

Another point that Neil stressed to me was the importance of not making The Talk sound like an apology. If you start out putting a negative spin on this topic, the other person is much more likely to react negatively. But if you can tell them in a matter-of-fact sort of way, then whether their reaction is positive or negative will be up to them.

> **Larry**—I met a guy I fell for and dinner-dated a few times, but without having sex. I remember sitting in his car one evening, telling him the Awful Truth (as I saw it). I must have sounded as though I was dying of something. He did not seem fazed about it, but he soon faded out of my life with no explanations, as some men do. I have no idea whether my herpes had anything to do with this.

Larry, in this example he cited, took the wrong approach, making it more of a big deal than it should be, and so he'll never know whether he turned off this particular man or not. But just the way first impressions count, the impression you give about having herpes will also count. If you make it seem as if you've been inflicted with a dreadful disease, then it's more likely that the person you're telling will believe you, especially if they don't know that much about herpes to begin with. And while I'm not advising you to put a positive spin on what you have, staying as neutral about it as possible will end up sending as positive a message as possible.

> **A.T.**—Do not be on the defensive, because that partner probably has something to say to you. If you're dealing with an adult partner, it's more than likely that individual has had some experience with some STD. Even if they don't have herpes, they may have chlamydia, gonorrhea, genital warts, etc. Make sure you discuss your entire sexual history so that this other person sees you're not promiscuous. Begin slowly and eventually a light will go off in their head and they'll see that you're right. And if you're a guy, remember you can't wait too long because if

you're not making a sexually aggressive move within a month or so, she's going to wonder what's going on.

While reiterating the concept of not being defensive about your herpes, A.T. adds an important point regarding timing. If herpes, or some other STD, weren't in the picture, a new relationship would proceed at a certain pace. If you're stalling because you're afraid of having The Talk, the other person is going to start to wonder what is going on. They may think that you're really not interested, or that you don't find them attractive. You could end up losing this potential partner before ever having the opportunity to talk to them about herpes, and that would be worse than losing them because of having herpes as then you'll never know what their reaction would have been. So while you don't need to bring it up on the first date, you also don't want to wait too long.

How to Have The Talk

Stephanie—I have had The Talk on quite a number of occasions. It isn't easy, but it helps me if I do this in the most open and honest way I can. My version of The Talk goes something like this:

"Listen, there's something very important I need to explain to you. Several years ago I was in a relationship, with a man I cared for deeply. Unfortunately, fidelity was not his 'best thing,' and he cheated on me. Even more unfortunate was the fact that in the process, he contracted herpes and gave it to me. I don't know how familiar you are with this virus"—then they usually tell me they know very little—"but I need you to fully understand the ramifications of this. Because it is a virus, it will always be with me—I can never be rid of it. I can control it to a great degree with antivirals, but I can never reduce the risk of transmission to zero. Current research seems to indicate that the likelihood of transmission while using antivirals and taking precautions is quite small, around 3 or 4 percent, but it is still a risk. So, I want you to have a clear understanding of the issue and make an informed decision, which I promise I will respect. I won't be angry, I won't be hurt, if you decide this is something you can't deal with. I wish someone had given me the opportunity to make an informed choice—I didn't get that, but you will. I'll e-mail you some information, and I'll answer any questions you have."

Other hints about having The Talk: While you don't have to have The Talk immediately (like as you sit down on your first date), you really do need to have it before you're in a difficult position (e.g., have it with all your clothes on). My personal opinion is that you also don't want to wait *too* long, because he may feel that he's been led on or betrayed. Do it in a quiet, private setting. Be calm and direct, and look him in the eye. Make sure you have additional information with you in print, or know where to find it online. Allow for the possibility that he may need some time to think, and let him know that whatever he decides, it's okay.

Stephanie offers very good advice, and she's obviously honed her skills each time she's had to have The Talk. That's something you can do too, even before you actually have The Talk. Neil suggests talking in front of a mirror. But others find a receptive audience at support groups.

Mark—If they have a new relationship and are about to have that certain conversation, they role-play with other group members. Not only do they get to practice, but they get feedback on their style. They also get to hear what happened to other group members when they've had The Talk and can learn from their mistakes.

I realize that not everyone who reads this book will be able to find a support group, which is one reason why you may have bought this book to begin with. But while support groups offer leaders who are very familiar with the subject, and are so very valuable in giving you feedback, that doesn't mean that because you're not part of a group you can't try out your Talk on some real live people. If you've already told some family and friends that you have herpes, then why not ask some of them to hear what you are going to say? Then listen to their criticisms. You don't have to accept them, but at least hear them out and then if they give you any tips that seem useful incorporate them into your Talk.

There is one disadvantage of doing this that I must point out. Many people go to a support group for only a limited amount of time and then they're on their own. But if you pull those closest to you into your love life, they're going to remain interested partners. Some people don't mind that, but if the risks of being rejected are made even stronger because you have herpes, then that might be a painful situation that you don't want to broadcast.

One way of getting around this dilemma is to practice having The Talk with some friends or relatives, but not make it specific to a particular upcoming Talk. Just say that you want to practice so that you'll be prepared if the moment ever arises. Tell them it will ease your mind if you can figure out what you're going to say way ahead of time. You can do this whether or not there actual is a Talk in your immediate future. This way you'll have the benefits of practicing without having to lose too much of your privacy.

Of course, if you have a close friend with whom you share every part of your life, then by all means engage in some role-playing in the period right before you're going to actually tell someone. I'm not saying that there is anything wrong with telling a close friend about your love life, but I do know that revealing such secrets is not everybody's cup of tea.

> **Anna**—I started thinking about how to tell him. I ran the gamut of factual information versus emotional story. I had the most intense anxiety I can imagine. I broke out in itchy bumps/hives and thought it was herpes all over me.

No matter how well prepared you are, you can't get away from the fact that having The Talk is going to be nerve-wracking, especially the first time. While you don't want to blow it up out of proportion, you also shouldn't try to minimize it. It's okay if you're nervous. Or even very nervous. There are some moments in this life in which having a case of nerves is unavoidable. It comes with the territory, as they say. But unless you have a bad heart, a severe case of nervousness won't kill you. You're not actually doing anything dangerous. It's like going on a roller coaster. Your stomach may be in a knot as the car inches its way up the first slope, but you're not actually in any danger. And people pay good money and stand on long lines to go on the very scariest roller coasters. So just because you're scared doesn't mean that you should give up. If you're successful, you might find true love and your life partner. And even if you don't get that lucky, you might find a partner for a limited amount of time.

Points to Cover

Obviously the story of how you got herpes is going to be at least somewhat different from those of other people, but when planning what you are going to say when having The Talk, there are some points that everyone needs to cover, so I want to go over these. I've placed them in a certain order, but you don't have to stick to the order I've selected. You don't even have to include each one of them, if you find that the individual you are talking to might react negatively to one of them. But this list will give you some guidelines to follow.

1. *I have herpes.* I've placed this first for an important reason. If you start having The Talk but you don't mention the disease, the person you are addressing may jump to the wrong conclusion. For example, they may think you are about to announce that you have AIDS. At that thought they may already have decided they want to have nothing more to do with you, and just because it turns out to be herpes instead of AIDS may not be enough to change their mind back again.

2. *It's not life-threatening.* When I talk to people about herpes, I find that many know very little about it except that it's not a good thing to have. They're not sure why it's not a good thing, and because of all the publicity AIDS has received, they might assume that like AIDS, herpes is deadly. You should disabuse them of that notion as soon as possible, as that idea could also cloud their brain so that they don't really hear the rest of what you have to say.

3. *As many as 60 million Americans have genital herpes.* If so many people have it, you are obviously not a freak for having caught it. Nor does it mean you've had sex with an untold amount of people. If the number of people you've had sex with is small, then come right out and tell them. In other words, let them know that this is a common disease and that you are not un-common for having caught it.

4. *It's incurable, contagious, but treatable.* One of the first thoughts to go through this person's mind will be: "If I have sex with them, am I going to get it?" You can't lie and say that you can guarantee that they won't, but you also have to let them know that by your taking the proper precautions, especially by tak-

ing the proper medication, the odds can be greatly reduced.
These low odds might still be too high for them, but you have
to let them know that having a sexual relationship with you
doesn't guarantee that they'll get herpes.

5. *Getting herpes may bring on a severe outbreak, but not necessarily
   so.* Even if you were to give a partner herpes, that doesn't mean
   that this person is going to have a severe case of herpes. Since
   statistically only 10 percent of people with herpes know they
   have it, that means that at least 90 percent of people who get
   it don't have a severe outbreak. And of the remaining 10
   percent who do know, not every one of them ever has a severe outbreak. You don't want to paint too rosy a picture because this person, having at least a vague image of herpes as
   being something dire, won't believe you, and then if that
   person does have sex with you and does get herpes, they'll be
   extra resentful because they'll think you led them on. Here's
   the moment when you probably should offer them some
   pamphlets so that they don't have to take your word for it
   but can see that the experts agree with what you are saying.

6. *Condoms alone cannot prevent anyone from getting herpes.* Because
   of AIDS our society has done a very good job of pushing
   condoms in order to have safe sex. First of all, I don't believe
   in using that term. Instead I use "safer sex," because even without herpes, condoms can break or fall off, so they're not 100
   percent foolproof when it comes to other diseases. And, as
   you already know, condoms can't give 100 percent protection against herpes because the virus may be shed from parts
   of the body not covered by a condom. It's important to say
   this because if this person decides not to form a relationship
   with you, he or she should know that they're at risk with any
   future partners they might have even if they use condoms.

7. *The bottom line is that at least with me, you know the risks and can
   take preventive action, but if you go back into the dating market-
   place, there are 60 million people out there who can also give you*

herpes but who can't warn you of the risks because they don't know they have the disease. Now I don't believe in scare tactics, and this is a scare tactic of sorts, but it's also the truth. If you're taking valacyclovir, which has now been shown to not only ease symptoms and prevent outbreaks, but also to prevent the transmission of the disease, you do offer less of a risk than a lot of other people who also have herpes but don't know it. I wouldn't expect anyone to accept this argument right away, but it is one that may slowly work its way into this potential partner's thinking if they need to justify to themselves why they should go ahead with this relationship.

I think after reading this chapter you have a better idea of how to have The Talk, but it's also still a pretty scary proposition. I certainly haven't offered you any guarantees that you won't be rejected, and that's true no matter how good you become at giving this Talk. But at the very least I hope that you now see a light at the end of the tunnel, and if you've been avoiding the dating scene up until now, that you'll be able to gather up your courage and go out and try to meet a new partner.

Chapter Highlights

1. The Talk may be nerve-wracking but it's not an impossible obstacle to finding a future partner.
2. Tell past partners so that they don't keep on spreading the disease.
3. Know the facts so that you can handle any questions that the other person poses.
4. Don't be negative or you're more likely to get a negative reaction.

6

Finding a Partner

As we all know, finding a partner is not the easiest thing in the world for many people. And the older we get, the harder it seems. When you are in school surrounded by other people your age, there are plenty of opportunities to meet potential partners, but when you're through with school, those opportunities can quickly evaporate. And with the fear of being accused of sexual harassment looming over the workplace, what should be a natural place to meet others has become much less so for those with full-time employment. Even if you do find a partner, considering that the divorce rate hovers around 50 percent, it's not necessarily a done deal even when you think you've found your mate for life. So at any given time, there are millions of single people looking to find Mr. or Ms. Right and not having all that much success.

Obviously this process is a lot more complicated if you have herpes. Notice I didn't say more *difficult*. It can be more difficult but it doesn't have to be, and one reason is that by having contracted herpes, you're now in a niche. I'm not saying that you have to look for a partner who also has herpes, but by narrowing down the field, it can make it easier. This does complicate the process also, but more on that later.

How Medications Are Changing the Process

At this point, I'm going to stick to those people with herpes who are not limiting themselves to one group, but considering the whole field. That's mostly because there is a major change coming to those who have herpes. The FDA has found that the drug valacyclovir has been shown to prevent the spread of herpes, as well as reduce the symptoms of those who have it. That means that someone with herpes who takes this drug daily can reduce the odds of his or her partner getting it to a great degree. It's not 100 percent effective but it is a significant reduction if on top of that you take every other precaution, the chances of transmitting it are actually quite minor. And, of course, any antiviral medication would also help reduce the severity of any symptoms a potential partner might have, if you were unlucky enough to pass on the disease. So that means that getting herpes is becoming a less scary proposition, which in turn means your disease won't scare people away to quite the same degree.

But while these changes are basically here, they suffer from obscurity. The effectiveness of this drug is not well known outside the community of those with herpes, and sadly, not that familiar to many people who do have herpes. And even with the possibilities opened up by this drug, there will continue to be residual fears to the word "herpes" for many years to come.

> **V.Y.W.**—After about eight months of not dating or seeing anyone, I went out with a guy and he was really really cruel with me. Face to face, he took it calmly and said he would think about it, but, later on the phone, he was rude and he was like, "How dare you talk to me!!" and "LOSE MY NUMBER!!" That type of deal.

What makes people act this way? Mostly it's ignorance. If they believe that herpes is a really terrible disease, and that it would severely change their lives if they got it, then they're going to overreact. And fear also has a role to play here. When you're afraid, adrenaline kicks in and you don't act normally. The fight-or-flight syndrome takes over and while eventually you might regret what you've done, at the moment your natural reaction is not to put the other person's feelings above your own.

> **Tanya**—I spent about a year and a half in total celibacy, mainly because I could not imagine telling anyone that I had herpes. The first guy I told was very compassionate but shied away from dating me. We're still friends to this day, and he insists that herpes was not the reason we did not continue dating, but he can't tell me exactly what it was, if anything.

And even if people don't overreact outwardly, you have no idea what is going on inside their heads. For example, in the case of Tanya's friend, there's no way to tell what he was thinking. Perhaps his decision was entirely based on Tanya's herpes, or maybe it was only part of the reason. But when you're rejected, the feeling is only slightly mitigated by having it done gently. It still is going to hurt, and rejection also makes it more difficult to go back out into the dating scene.

> **Tanya**—After that, every guy I told, for over twelve years, accepted me, and did not let herpes stop them from dating me. Life was great.

Tanya didn't let this one man's reaction stop her from pushing forward with her search, and you shouldn't either. Rejection is part of the game: the dating game and the game of life. You can't allow yourself to become paralyzed by the risks, because the rewards are too good to pass up.

A.E.—I met a man at a party and we started dating. After a while I said, "I have something to tell you," while we were cuddling in bed. I had been putting it off and didn't want to be rejected. I ended up crying, but he had a girlfriend who had it and he didn't get it and so he didn't reject me. That was an important step, realizing that a man won't necessarily reject me because I have herpes. I thought of myself as being tainted but that didn't mean everyone else did too.

If you go around thinking of yourself as tainted, as having that scarlet *H* on your forehead, that is definitely going to make it more difficult to find a partner. As you well know, when you're first dating, you look at the other person very carefully. You don't know them yet and you try to figure out what makes them tick. Because of this scrutiny, minor faults can appear to be major ones. Things you overlook in other people become unacceptable in this person. And so if he or she is giving off vibes that there is something wrong, you're going to sense that and maybe make more of a big deal about it than you would if you knew what it was. That's why it's important to have as much self-control about your herpes as possible. Yes, even if you break down and cry it's possible this potential partner won't be driven away. But some would be, and your job is to minimize those risks.

It's at this stage that you have to lean on that silver lining. You have to say to yourself, "Yes, I'm going to bare part of my soul by telling this person that I have herpes, but how he or she reacts to this information is going to tell me a lot about them. They may judge me because of my herpes, but I'm going to see what they're made of by how they react to this news." To whatever degree is possible, you have to consider yourself a cool scientist conducting an experiment. You're going to make yourself vulnerable, it's true, but you're also going to be making some discoveries. Think of yourself as a deep-sea diver looking for exotic fish. Yes, it's a bit scary diving down into deep waters, but when you find a particularly rare specimen, nothing is more exciting.

Permit me to carry this diving metaphor one step further. In the old days, divers wore big heavy suits and they were attached to the ship via a long oxygen line. On their head they wore giant headgear with only a small glass pane to see out of. Obviously their vision was severely limited. Then scuba tanks were invented and people could dive while looking all around them. Their ability to see the various forms of sea life grew enormously.

There are many people who look for a partner while wearing one of those old diving rigs—metaphorically, that is. They carry so much psychological baggage that they pass up most people they meet. And certainly the guilt, pain, and shame of herpes can be a part of that. But if you can free yourself of these constraints, then the pool of people who might be suitable opens up and your odds of finding someone increase too.

Jane—The dilemma now is always do I wait until I'm emotionally involved with someone to tell them, then if it's a big issue and they walk away, which is a choice I respect, I end up hurt. That has happened to me. Or do I tell them up front before we know each other that well to spare my own broken heart if it is an issue with them. I've done both.

There's a classic episode of *Seinfeld* that dealt with the removal of the contraceptive sponge from the market. Elaine and some other women preferred using the sponge and so stocked up on all they could get their hands on. Then it was a question of deciding whether or not a man was "sponge-worthy"—in other words, would having sex with this man be worth dipping into their cache of contraceptive sponges?

People with herpes face a similar decision. It's hard to have The Talk, no matter how many times you've done it before, and so you have to weigh the worth of having it or not. As I said before, it makes casual sex harder, which may be a good thing. But if you wait until you are emotionally involved to have The Talk, then it makes being rejected, if that's what is going to happen, that much harder to accept also. So there's a decision you have to make at some point whether or not this person is "Talk-worthy." And it seems to me that it's better to make that decision sooner rather than later and to get The Talk over and done with so that if it turns out that the relationship will not develop, then you won't have wasted too much time with this person.

Does The Talk Have to Lead to Sex?

At this point I must deal with an important question: Does having The Talk mean that you have to have sex soon after? As you know, I'm in favor of there being a relationship before you have sex with someone. But I've also just said that you shouldn't wait too long to have The Talk, because if things don't work out, you don't want to have wasted too much time on this person. If you have The Talk, though, doesn't that then mean that sex is imminent?

I realize that some people may think that way, but it doesn't have to be. For example, I encourage parents to talk to their children about sex. Certainly once children are physically capable of having sex—by their early teens, say—parents need to make certain that they understand how sex works. But that doesn't mean, by any stretch of the imagination, that by telling their children about sex they want them to go out and engage in it. In fact, when they give this instruction it is also a perfect opportunity to explain to them why they should wait to have sex until they're older.

The same theory holds true when having The Talk. At the same time that you're telling this person that you have herpes, you can certainly also tell them that just because you have herpes does not mean that you are promiscuous and that you don't have sex with people you are dating until the relationship has developed to a certain point. Your timetable for getting to the stage when sex is acceptable is something this person was going to find out anyway, perhaps more in a hit-and-miss sort of way amid the fumbling that couples often go through. You can be certain that he or she was curious as to this point, and was thinking about it just as much as you were. So having this discussion will clear the air and maybe end up being just as much a relief for this other person as getting it out of the way is for you.

Of course, there are some people who don't want to wait to have sex, whether or not herpes is involved. So you might lose some potential partners after this discussion not because you have herpes, but because you won't jump into the sack on the second or third date. But again, that's a silver lining. If the two of you have a great difference in this arena, it's better for both of you to find out as soon as possible so that you don't waste time in the early stages of a relationship that is not going anywhere.

There's one more silver lining that I haven't talked about yet, and that's the fact that having The Talk changes a relationship in a good way. You can be much more open with each other after having had The Talk. This, in turn, means that you should be able to communicate more easily about how to have sex. For example, if a woman needs certain caresses in order to have an orgasm, she'll have an easier time confiding the secrets of her arousal to a partner with whom she's already had an intimate discussion than one with whom the conversations have been on a more superficial level.

This is a very important point, so let me go into it a bit more. Each sex has one sexual problem that is shared by many of its members. Many women have difficulties having an orgasm, and many of those just fake it rather than tell their partner that they need this or that in order to arrive at sexual satisfaction. Many men suffer from premature ejaculation. Dealing with PE is not that difficult if both partners work at it together, but often that doesn't happen and the couple ignores the problem, rather than deal with it, and sometimes end up breaking up over it, even though it was never mentioned. (Or perhaps is gets mentioned in fights rather than in constructive behavior.)

But if a couple has established a certain degree of intimacy by having The Talk, it should make it much easier to talk about any sexual problems they may have, and then fix them. As I said, these two common problems are not without solutions, but they require cooperation between the two parties. So by establishing better communications by having The Talk, issues of sexual dysfunction, be they mild or major, can then be more easily dealt with.

So don't look at having to wait to have The Talk until you're just about at the point of having sex. You don't want to have it on a first or second date, while you're still making up your mind whether this person is worth pursuing, but you also don't have to wait until the last second. You might as well enjoy the benefits of The Talk as soon as possible, so don't make the mistake of putting it off until the last moment.

Finding a Partner

Before you even get to this stage, you have to find someone to actually date, which is the topic of this chapter. (I bet you thought I would never get here, right? Sorry, sometimes I wander but there's so much to say that it can be difficult to get straight to the point.) As I said earlier, I'm going to deal first with dating in general, before getting to specific suggestions for people with herpes.

The most important key to successful dating is to be open to the process. For every barrier that you put up, the degree of difficulty goes up. For example, assume you say that you won't go to bars to meet people, but you do go to bars with your friends now and then. Well, when you're at that bar, you should be ready, willing, and able to meet someone if the opportunity presents itself. And even if it doesn't, if you see someone who looks appealing and is not with someone, do whatever it takes to meet them.

Not going to bars is just one of the many barriers that people put up. Some insist on a certain level of income. Or that the other person went to the right school. Or drives a certain car. Or has looks that are acceptable according to some artificially numbered rating system. If you're the type of person who never had any problem meeting people who met your criteria before you had herpes, maybe you'll be just as lucky afterward. But it's also possible that you won't have the same success. At that point, you'll have to change your standards, which may also be a silver lining because there are probably plenty of people out there who would make you very happy even though they fail one or more of the tests you've been using.

The Bar Scene

Okay, so you've decided not to turn down any opportunity to meet a new partner, even someone you meet at a bar. Since meeting people is an active rather than a passive process, you're going to have to take some action rather than just sit there like a lump. But whatever you do, don't make the mistake of going about the process of trying to meet this stranger out of desperation or by coming on too strong. That's going to give them the wrong message. You may need to use some "come-on" line, but it should be a subtle one.

My advice is to start with eye contact, and if that seems to be leading somewhere, then pick yourself up and go over and say, "Hi, my name is . . . " (This is particularly important if you're with a group, which might seem intimidating to a stranger.) Your next line, after this person says "Hi" back and gives you his or her name, is an important one. It shouldn't be cheesy or you'll look bad. You shouldn't try to be witty, as the joke might fall flat. I would suggest it be a question, as that will automatically lead to a response, and it should be a question that the other person can answer easily. A very good one is "What do you do when you're not here in this bar?" Hopefully they won't say something witty back but will give you a simple answer about their job, something they ought to know a lot about. At that point you can either ask more questions about them, or if they ask you about your line of work, which they probably will if they're not tongue-tied, you can answer their question.

After several minutes of casual banter, you should have some idea whether or not you have any interest in pursuing this person. If you do, you could invite him or her back to join your friends, or just keep on talking right at the bar. If you want to go back to your friends, you could ask that person for a phone number or e-mail address. (I would advise you to carry some small blank cards that you can write on. That way you can decide at that moment how much information you want to give out. If you give someone your business card, that might contain more information than you want to make known at that point.)

Of course, the reverse may happen and someone may come up to you. Don't judge someone only by their opening remarks or the way they look. It's not easy to start up a conversation with a stranger. Just because the first few sentences someone utters are cheesy does not mean that the person is a cheese. And also realize that some of the men with the best pick-up lines are exactly the type of person that you don't want to be associated with, because all they're interested in is a one-night stand. And the women showing the most cleavage may be the ones who are the least likely to be someone you'd want to wake up with every morning. So gather as much information as you can before reacting. Look for those diamonds in the rough. They're not always easy to spot but the reward is well worth it.

Another important aspect of meeting people in bars is to control your intake of alcohol. If you're out with friends with no interest in finding a mate, then you can drink a bit more heavily, but if your judgment is impaired, that's not likely to be helpful if you are looking to find a partner. After you've had a real drink, switch to a soft drink that can look as if it has alcohol in it, or a nonalcoholic brand of beer, and pour it in a glass. Then later on you can have another real drink. Too many people have gone off with someone they met at a bar when drunk and later regretted it, especially women who were raped.

Don't be afraid to bring props to the bar. It could be a hat or T-shirt from somewhere exotic (where you've been or at least have a story about). It could be a magazine or book (though not the *Kama Sutra!*). Wear a pin of some sort that looks interesting. Or bring along a little digital camera. Take some pictures of your friends and the flash will draw the attention of those around you. Someone may then comment on your camera just as an excuse to make conversation. And if you take a picture of them, you can then ask for their e-mail address so that you can send it to them.

Try not to stay rooted to one spot. If you're imbibing alcohol, especially beer, you'll definitely have to go to the toilet at some point, but don't be afraid to walk around by yourself at other times. Your friends will still be there as an anchor, but if you make yourself a little vulnerable by separating yourself from time to time, you'll be more likely to make connections with other people who might be hesitant to approach an entire group of people. This might not occur the first time or two that you go for such a stroll, but who knows about the third or fourth?

And most importantly, don't let yourself get discouraged. If you've had some good laughs with your friends, the night wasn't a total loss just because you failed to meet anyone interesting. Always try to make the best of each situation. There will be a highlight film of your life, but just because this one episode didn't include any doesn't mean that it wasn't worth living.

I've made this sound simple, and it is. What's difficult is when you zero in on someone and you bomb out. In other words, you may be rejected. That's a hard thing to accept, especially if your friends are witnesses to it. But while it's hard, it's not impossible, and so it's a risk that you must take.

Analyzing Rejection

What if you try over and over again and you're always rejected? I know that you're not a virgin, since you have herpes, so that means you connected with at least one other person. That should always give you hope. I get letters from young people who've never had a date and they can be desperate, and if the other person feels that you're desperate, that will surely turn them off. But if you're striking out again and again, even if you did once have a partner, it's time for some analysis.

The first thing I would suggest is to ask your friends what you're doing wrong. Don't get mad at them and don't automatically reject what they have to say, either, but listen carefully and try to make some adjustments. For example, if enough people tell you that you're not dressed fashionably, then if finding a partner is important to you, you have to make some changes in your wardrobe. You don't have to go out and buy an entire new wardrobe, unless your clothes are all ten years old. Perhaps just getting a new shirt or top would be enough to make a difference. Try that and see what happens. Then you can keep making these small adjustments until you've hit the point where you're becoming more successful.

You might also learn a valuable lesson from this experience. You might have resisted the old adage that clothes make the man. You might have been saying to yourself, "People should like me for who I am, not what I wear." But if you then see that people are reacting to your clothes, rather than fighting reality, you should give in to it. Sometimes in life you just have to admit that you're wrong.

Now there are some things about you that you cannot change. I, for example, never grew past 4'7", and being short is just something I had to learn to accept. Just as there are people who might reject you because you have herpes, there are going to be people who will reject you because of your height, your girth, whether your hair is curly or straight, or the size of your nose. *C'est la vie,* as the French say. What you have to hold on to is the fact that if you try your hardest to look your best, there are people out there who would be willing to be your partner. But if you have some natural problems with your appearance, and on top of that you don't try to make yourself look your best, then it's quite likely that you will spend a lot of time alone.

A Dose of Realism

In addition to making the most of your appearance, whatever it is, the other tool you need to date successfully is a dose of realism. While it would be great if everybody could find somebody who looked like a top model to date, the fact is that there aren't enough of them to go around. The same would hold true of people with great intelligence and great wealth. In other words, you're probably going to have to make some compromises vis-à-vis your fantasy lover. Some people don't know how to accept that fact of life. They constantly try to connect with someone who has all the characteristics they seek in an ideal mate. Since none of these people are perfect themselves, it's not surprising that they fail time and time again.

I once had a young lady ask me to introduce her to a very famous comedian. Even if I could have done this, I certainly would not have invaded his privacy this way. But more important, this young lady, while very nice, was just not going to be able to beat out all the women who were after this comedian. She had an unrealistic dream, and she spent her nights alone because of it. Sadly she is not alone in falling into this trap.

In seeking a partner, the most important traits someone can offer you are companionship, good conversation, an open mind, and hopefully love and sexual arousal. Anything else is just icing on the cake. And if looks are the most important quality you desire in a partner, then don't be surprised if you wind up in a never-ending search because even if you do succeed in finding someone who is interested in you who is very good-looking, you're probably going to run into other people who are even better-looking and you'll be off to the chase once again. It's very difficult to sate an appetite based solely on looks, so most people who get caught up in this game wind up constantly playing but never winning.

Tell the World

Another way of being open to the process is to admit to everyone you know that you're looking for a partner. That includes friends, family, coworkers, and anyone else you know who might be able to set you up. If you have two hundred people on your buddy list, let them all know you're looking. There's no shame in letting people know that you're interested in finding a partner. In the Jewish faith, making a match is a good deed, and most people would enjoy helping someone find true love. If there's anyone who thinks you're being foolish, then they're not a real friend and it doesn't matter what they think.

The reason that I'm suggesting you let as many people know as possible is that this will increase the odds of success. If you let only ten people know, there may be no one in that group who knows someone else of the opposite sex who would be right for you. But once the number starts to grow, so do the odds.

Again, I don't want you to sound desperate. You have to convince them what a great catch you are. (Maybe not close relatives, but everybody else.) Tell these people what type of person it is you're looking for, so that no one tries to set you up with someone who is absolutely wrong for you. But don't give indications that you're too choosy, or the people you tell this to won't even bother trying. It may take you a while to develop the right approach, one that will make the people you contact want to help you without feeling sorry for you. It can be hard to be honest about yourself, so maybe you want to work on this with a close friend or two. They'll be able to tell you whether your tone sounds like you're bragging, which might turn people off, or if you're not doing a good enough job of building yourself up. It's a balancing act, but not one so difficult that you can't figure it out, especially with the help of others.

You may have to go through this procedure more than once. First of all, some of the people you contact will be so busy that they'll forget about your request, even if they happen to know just the right person. And as time goes by, others will learn of people who are looking for a partner whom they didn't know about when you first put the word out. So if the first go-round doesn't pan out, don't abandon this method, because it can yield results.

One result of this type of broadcasting is going to be blind dates, some of which could be disastrous. By "disastrous" I mean that you go out with someone whom you would never want to go out with again. The one good thing about blind dates is that at least someone knows this other person, so such dates are unlikely to lead to a dangerous situation. But the damage caused by such dates can be mitigated by proper planning. Say you wanted to try out a certain new restaurant or see a particular movie. If you can steer a blind date toward a place or activity that you're interested in, then you'll get something out of the time spent even if you don't ever see that person, at least willingly, again.

Blind dates are a hit-or-miss operation, but part of the reason might be because of people's expectations. The other person, who has been screened by a friend or relative, probably isn't really awful, but if that person has been built up, it might be difficult for him or her to live up to the picture that's been painted of them. And even if you've been given a realistic picture, you might still have high hopes that can come crashing down. My suggestion is to withhold judgment of this other person as long as possible. Try to keep an open mind and really look for this person's good points rather than allowing yourself to be distracted by any bad ones they may have. Go out of your way to be fair, rather than leaning the other way, stigmatizing this person because he or she is a blind date. Remember, you're also a blind date, and you're not perfect either. I know that even if you maintain the best of intentions, the odds of a blind date working out are not that high, but do what you can to increase them rather than lower them.

One thing you should not do is broadcast to everyone you know that you're going on a blind date. Your friends are going to want to know how it went and this almost forces you to make up your mind very quickly. If you're looking across the table at this person as if all your friends were at your shoulder looking too, then it's going to be much harder to be quite as discerning as you might be. It's possible that you might not be able to tell on only one date, but if your friends know you're going on a second date, then they might make more of it than it's worth, and so you might even skip that second date if it's going to be public. So tell the friend who sets you up to keep their mouth shut, and you do the same; that will remove a lot of the pressure from this sort of situation and therefore make a positive outcome much more likely.

Take Action

But you can't only rely on the goodwill of others. You have to put yourself into situations where you might meet someone. I suggest that you plan certain activities that you find interesting and that might also lead to meeting potential dating partners. Let's say you enjoy going to museums and would like to learn more about art.

Taking a class at a museum would be a way of sating that particular thirst for knowledge, while at the same time it would put you into a situation where you'd be meeting new people. Such classes are no-lose propositions because you'll get something out of taking them no matter what. You might also meet someone to date, or even someone who just becomes a good friend, so there is a definite upside to this sort of activity.

If you're in the hunt for a mate, and there are several courses or activities that you might have an interest in, it goes without saying that you should choose the one where you are most likely to meet a potential partner. For example, if you're a woman and like quilting and tennis, head for the tennis courts before you sign up for any quilting classes.

An Admonition

And don't tell me that there are no courses that appeal to you that would also appeal to the opposite sex! Once you start making excuses, then you're saying loud and clear you're really not that eager to find someone. But if it is a high priority, then there really are no excuses. I understand that some parts of this process are not under your control, but so much of this process *is* under your control that you could fill your days and nights actively searching. But if all you're doing is sitting by the phone waiting for it to ring, and you haven't put out any feelers in order to induce those rings, then I can't take you seriously, and if you don't find a partner, don't blame me.

Other Places to Look

Classes aren't the only place to look for a member of the opposite sex. Places of worship often have other activities, including dances, concerts, and potluck suppers, that may be a good place to look. Many people go to certain shops, like bookstores, in order to browse the aisles for more than just the merchandise that's for sale. There are always social events taking place and while some are mostly for couples, there are many that might also be appropriate places to look for a partner. These might cost you some money for a ticket, but since many of these are to benefit a charity, you can never look at it as a waste. And even the time you spend commuting might be a good place to be on the lookout for a potential date, though that doesn't apply if you drive. But if you take public transportation, and tend to go and return at the same time every day, you're likely to see other people regularly. If any look appealing, and aren't wearing wedding rings, then you might find an excuse to strike up a conversation and see what develops. And if one time, or one specific car on the train, doesn't bear fruit, try another.

The Importance of Body Language

Many people who ride public transportation have a scowl on their face. If it's early and they're heading for work, perhaps you can't blame them for looking miserable, but if everyone else has a sour puss, that's all the more reason for you to wear a smile. Having a bright attitude will make you stand out, so even if you smile at a much older person near you, that might give a positive impression to someone your age who's sitting a few feet away.

You'll also find many commuters with their eyes occupied, either reading or closed. But if you look around, you might be able to lock eyes with an attractive person of the opposite sex. That's the time to flash your smile and see what response you get. If it seems positive, then if you try to strike up a conversation, there's a better than even chance that your efforts will be rewarded. Knowing ahead of time that the other person is going to be receptive makes initiating further contact so much easier. So pay attention to your body language when you're in a public place and make sure that you're giving off positive vibes that will be attractive to the opposite sex.

"But Dr. Ruth," I hear some of you women saying right now, "what if I look right into the eyes of a geek?" While many men try to catch women's eyes, many women do all they can to avoid such eye contact because they're afraid that some "geek" or "nerd" will come over and bother them. To my way of thinking, if you're single and looking to find a partner, that's not an attitude you can afford. So what if someone you don't want to date comes up to you? First of all, they're paying you a compliment. They're saying that they find you attractive. Instead of looking at that as a negative, look at it as a positive. And then, if you've had a string of bad relationships, maybe you should try going out with someone who's not that great-looking but who would be loyal and attentive. If someone is dressed like a slob, something under their control, I can understand not wanting to be associated with them. But if their looks aren't that great because of what Mother Nature gave them, then perhaps they have other qualities that may not be so apparent but that far outweigh their looks. So be more open to the idea of looking beyond appearances.

In any case, if you're going to act very guarded whenever you're in public, then you're cutting yourself off from many possible Mr. Rights. I say to be more accepting of having men approach you, even those who you are certain are not your type, in exchange for increasing the possibility that someone who is acceptable will be among them.

Finding the Love of Your Life Online

Millions of single people have registered themselves on one or more websites to further their search for a partner, and many have found success. I have to be honest and tell you that at first I had serious reservations about this entire process. I feel that it was too easy for someone to hide their real identity online and that meeting someone in this manner, particularly for a woman, was far too risky. While I'm sure there are still some perverts lurking around out there, the numbers of people using these services has grown so large, and the security precautions taken by many of these services have become so much more sophisticated, that it appears that the dangers are not much greater than those that also exist in meeting someone at a bar or through some other means.

The one factor that dating services share with every other method of meeting people is that they are still only a first step. The idea of purely virtual dating is just not appealing, and I hope it never will be. You want to be able to see and eventually touch this other person, and so at some point the computer will have to be moved aside and you'll have to meet. So it's really a matter of looking at an online dating service as just one more method of making that first step. There may be a slightly different skill set that you need to do this successfully, but since everything starts out very anonymously, it's no big deal if you make some initial mistakes while you're figuring it all out.

Dating Within the Herpes Community

So far in this chapter I've been treating people with herpes and those without on an equal footing. Obviously you have to meet people in order to get to the point where you're going to have The Talk, which I've already covered, so most of the time there is not much difference in the very early stages. But online dating is one area where people with herpes can separate themselves right from the beginning, as there are some online dating services that have been set up to serve only people who have herpes.

Ever since I got into the advice-giving business, I've been sent questions from people who have encountered great difficulties meeting people of the opposite sex, many because of their fear of being rejected. I've had some success in getting people to overcome this fear, which means I've gotten them to gather up their courage and take chances. That's why having people with herpes become dependent on the crutch of a herpes-only dating service does give me some concern, from a psychological perspective. But I also know that when someone breaks a leg, they require a crutch to get around at first, so hopefully anyone using such a service who doesn't find a partner will eventually be able to make the transition to using other methods of meeting people who don't necessarily have herpes.

Obviously if two people meet on a herpes-only online dating service, a major barrier is lifted. Instead of having to dread having The Talk, they can instead breathe a huge sigh of relief because this sword of Damocles isn't hanging over them. Of course, that's not entirely true. They may not have to talk about herpes, but HIV and the other STDs are still a risk factor that should be considered. Let's face it though: If you've admitted to someone that you have one STD, it becomes much less of a big deal to get tested for the others.

If the pool of people with herpes was very small, I might say that while it's all right to look in that community, you'll almost definitely have to expand your horizons beyond it. But I spoke with Anthony, who began MPwH, the largest online dating service for people with herpes, and he told me that they have about 40,000 registered members. That's not anywhere near as big as the behemoths of the industry, like Match.com, which has millions of registrants, but it's big enough that if you can't find someone among a group of that size to date, then you're going to have trouble finding someone through any other dating service as well.

Anthony explained that a site like MPwH offers other benefits besides opportunities to meet potential partners. He told me that his site also serves as a community where people with herpes could meet simply as friends, either strictly online or eventually in person. That's an added bonus to being part of a group like this, which you wouldn't find on one of the larger dating services, and I think it could be an important one. If you're not sure whether online dating is for you, you could get started by just looking around the site, and then, hopefully, meet someone interesting with whom you could further develop a relationship. But you'd know that even if you didn't meet anyone who was just right for you, you could definitely make some friends. If you've been having a hard time talking about herpes with your friends and family, you wouldn't be so constrained with this group of friends, and talking about your problems is certainly an important part of the recovery process.

As we've seen, there are some people who become absolutely immobilized by getting herpes. Just about everyone who gets herpes has an initial period where they are devastated by the news, but most people eventually move on from that point. Some, however, just can't seem to make those first steps. Having to reveal that they have herpes to a stranger is just not a situation with which they believe they can cope. For people in this group, getting herpes can be a condemnation to a lifetime of loneliness. Psychological counseling might be of service to them, but if they've retreated far into their shell, they might not even consider counseling as an option. And if they haven't even told their friends and family why they never go out on dates, then they lose even the psychological shoring up that this group could provide. So for those stuck in this particular jail, online dating services that cater to those with herpes are a lifesaver.

But as I said, since anyone with herpes has some trepidation when it comes to returning to the dating scene, *no one* with the disease should rule out these services, at least just to get your feet wet. Maybe you'll get lucky and find someone acceptable who has herpes, but even if you're more picky, going out on a few dates will give a boost to your confidence in your overall ability to date, so that if you later decide to look outside this particular pool to find a partner, it will be easier for you and you'll be more likely to meet with success.

I know that online dating services have existed for many years, and also know that literally millions of people use them, but I still want to throw in my two cents when it comes to taking the proper precautions. Even though I don't know you, believe me when I say I worry about you. Since I've given you my permission to use one of these services, if something were to happen to you, I'd feel very, very bad.

One problem with the longevity of this form of dating is that the people who prey on others have had a chance to become better at it. As the pool of potential victims has grown, those who try to take advantage of lonely people have become more sophisticated in the way they operate. They've got their stories down pat, and they've figured out what to say to counter your doubts about them. Nevertheless, they're still pushing a scam of some sort, so if you keep your wits about you, you should be able to learn to spot trouble.

I'm a great believer in trusting your instincts. If you sense any red flags, my advice is to stop having any contact with this person as soon as possible. What type of things could the other person say that might raise a red flag? If they brag about having lots of money, or maybe about being a member of the FBI or the Secret Service. If all their relatives have conveniently passed away. That may sound sad but it could just be part of their cover-up.

Of course, for you to be able to cut yourself off from this person means that they should not have a way of contacting you. That's why it's extremely important to follow whatever security guidelines the online dating service provides, especially with regard to revealing any real information about yourself. Make sure you have a separate screen name set up somewhere, like on hotmail, that can't be connected to you. Never give out your phone number. If you must give any type of number, make it a pager. But remember that these days, because of Caller ID, you have to be careful even if you are the one making the call. If you might be in a position to have to call someone who's basically a stranger, make sure that you've activated a Caller ID blocking feature so that no one can see the number of the person who is calling. Or else use a public phone. If you get to the point where you decide to meet, make it someplace very public, and not necessarily in your hometown. If you live in a big city, then it could be somewhere else in that city, but if you live in a small town, don't meet there. Don't even talk about your small town, but only mention the region.

I know it's sad to have to think this way. You don't want to be so suspicious, and because of that reluctance, it's easy to let your guard down. But you have to keep in mind that anyone who contacts you who does have bad intentions knows very well that a nice person can be induced to reveal information because of this reluctance to sound mean. It's one of those catch-22 situations, but for your own protection, you have to assume the worst in the other person for a certain amount of time. I can't tell you how long, but really can only repeat that you must trust your instincts and also err on the side of caution.

You might want to rely on more than one set of instincts. Even if you are not admitting that you are desperate, if deep down inside you're a little bit desperate, you might be willing to overlook certain things about a potential partner. You needn't be ashamed of such a reaction; it's perfectly natural. But while you shouldn't be ashamed of it, you also shouldn't ignore it. That's why asking a good friend's opinion of the facts that you know about this other person might be a good idea. Also, if you're going to meet, make sure that somebody else knows about this meeting, including where it is supposed to happen. You might want to have them call you on your cell phone a few times to make sure you're okay.

Do all these precautions sound a bit exaggerated? Perhaps to someone who never had anything ill befall them, but if you're reading this book the odds are that some person whom you didn't suspect of having herpes gave it to you. Therefore you, of all people, should be a bit more suspicious than you once were. So even if it seems petty to be so careful, it's better to go the extra mile than to have something else to regret later on.

Don't Give Up Hope

I can't end this chapter on such a bleak note. Yes, dating can be complicated, and sometimes even ugly, but there can also be high points. It's really one of those glasses that can be looked at as half empty or half full. And since how you look at dating will affect how successful you are, your attitude is key. So always try to think positively, whether you're still looking for a date or are actively dating. I'm certain you know somebody who you never thought would get married who did, even if very late in life. There is hope for anyone; the more you hold on to that hope, the more likely that it will help you make just the right connection.

Chapter Highlights

1. Having The Talk doesn't mean that you'll have sex, but it will help to clear the air.
2. Broadcast to everyone you know that you're looking.
3. Take action so that you won't miss out on any opportunities.
4. Maintain a positive attitude.

7

Living with Herpes as a Couple

W hile herpes may split up some relationships, it also becomes part of many others. In some cases both partners have the disease, while in others it's only one who has it. Herpes will have effects that need to be dealt with in either of these situations, and if you happen to fall into one of these, I want to offer you some advice on what you can do to make certain that herpes doesn't negatively affect your relationship.

When Both Have It

You might think that herpes wouldn't play much of a role in a couple where both partners have the disease, but there are definitely issues that can crop up. If a couple has a before-and-after-herpes history, there may be issues of trust. If one partner gave it to the other, there may be lingering doubts as to the circumstances. Many couples stay together after a crisis, but like a piece of shattered pottery that has been glued back together, the cracks may still be visible and they're also points of weakness. If one person is still harboring resentment toward the other about having been given herpes, that could change the entire nature of the relationship. Conversely, a person who gave herpes to his or her partner may stay in a relationship out of guilt, but that sort of relationship isn't a very strong one. So as you can see, there are potential pitfalls, most of which can be avoided if you remain on the alert.

Herpes Is Always with You

Many couples endure a crisis or two during the course of a long-term relationship, but usually the cause remains in the past. That is to say, after the crisis has occurred, it may leave a bad taste but it does not continue to show itself otherwise. But because there is no cure for herpes, any herpes-related issues between two people are going to show up again and again. Even if someone never has another outbreak because they're on suppressive therapy, each time they swallow a pill, they're going to be reminded of what happened. Any time that one person feels a herpes attack coming on, he or she may experience the same effect. And a real outbreak may cause an even more serious emotional crisis. It's because of herpes' ever-present nature that a couple has to be ever-vigilant.

When a sign of herpes, like a lesion for example, triggers an emotion, you can't stop yourself from having this particular emotional reaction. If it's going to make you angry or sad, you will feel that emotion, however intensely. But while that initial emotional response is not under your control, what happens after that is. Let's say you feel some itching that you recognize as prodome, a precursor of a herpes attack. You dash for the medicine cabinet and take an antiviral to fend off the effects of the disease, which probably will do the trick. But part of the anger you first felt at your partner for giving you herpes slithers into your consciousness. What's the best way of dealing with this anger?

Some people enjoy getting angry. They actually savor this emo-tion; once that fire is lit, they will try to feed it so that it grows even bigger. But anger aimed at your partner for something he or she did years ago is not healthy for your relationship, to put it mildly. And even worse is showing anger over a mere trifle that is really the re-sult of the anger you feel over the past, which your partner has no way of guessing. If you want to nourish your love for each other instead of basking in the red heat of that anger, what you must do is make a conscious effort to tamp it back down.

The simplest way you could accomplish this is to go to your partner, tell him or her that you had to take a pill to prevent an outbreak of herpes, and ask for a hug. Linger in your partner's arms for a few moments, and there's a good chance that when you pull away, your anger will have dissipated. Such a display of your love for each other will have allowed you to beat back the danger as a team, which is really the best way.

A hug may not do the trick for you but exactly how you deal with these type of emotions isn't all that important—you have to work out the best way of handling this. What is vital to the state of your relationship is that you do act to defend it from these emo-tional outbursts, or the damage they do each and every time will accumulate and eventually could destroy the partnership.

Don't Try to Bury Emotions

The first line of attack is to acknowledge the emotions that well up, or else you won't be able to counteract them. That's an important point that I want to stress. If each time you feel that anger or sad-ness you simply shrug it off, it may end up festering. At some later date, all these accumulated emotions may mutate into one giant emo-tional outburst that will be so strong you won't be able to ignore it. At that point maybe you'll start screaming at your partner over nothing or your partner will find you curled up in a chair sobbing, and he or she won't understand what's going on. In fact, you might not understand either. You might not grasp, at that particular moment, that the reason for this seeming overreaction is the accumulation of past emotions that you tried to bury. And one of these outbursts can then do lasting damage to your relationship. Compare it to a series of thunderstorms, which may be noisy but won't damage your house, and a hurricane, which can knock it to the ground. While you can't control the weather, you can prevent an emotional hurricane by taking care of the thunderstorms.

Of course, this job is one that you have to do together. It's not just the person undergoing these emotions who bears all the responsibility for defusing these situations. His or her partner has to be especially understanding and willing to give of themselves at these times. It will help this person if they understand that the emotions are not really directed against them. Yes, maybe he gave her herpes, but if she's feeling angry at a particular moment because of some sign of herpes, it doesn't mean that she's still angry with him. She loves him, and the anger is more of a general anger at life. (If she's still harboring a huge chip on her shoulder toward him, then that's another, more serious problem.) If he acts defensively, she may then turn her anger at him, but that doesn't have to happen. If he just gives her a sympathetic ear, allows himself to act as a sounding board for her anger for a few minutes without reacting, the storm will pass and hopefully everything will be back to normal.

I'm not saying that it's easy to take this sort of "punch." If someone is angry and it appears that this anger might be directed at you, or even something you caused, then your defenses are likely to spring into action. It takes an act of will to bring them back down. You must allow your brain to rule your emotions at moments like these. You have to remind yourself how much you love your partner and how much the relationship means to you.

It also takes practicing the art of communication. She has to let him know that this particular outbreak of anger is being caused by herpes, not because he left his socks on the floor for the umpteenth time. (That's also a problem that needs to be fixed, but that's not within the scope of this book.) But if she lets him know that her anger is herpes-related, then he has to be able to cut her some slack when it comes to his reaction, and hopefully, because they are both working toward a peaceful resolution, within a few moments, the crisis will have passed.

By the way, I'm suggesting that the partner join this battle not out of guilt, but rather out of love. If you can both act as a team to fight a common enemy—in this case, the emotions caused by herpes—then your relationship will actually end up stronger. Another one of those silver linings, I suppose. So make sure that you sit down and talk about your reactions to herpes, figure out how you can each help the other, and then carry out your plan of action as consistently as possible.

Of course, there will be exceptions. If one of you has had a particularly bad day at the office, for example, that person might not be able to react calmly to an emotional outburst on the home front. Nobody's perfect and we all have to adapt to circumstances. But if you do the best you can to rise to the occasion most of the time, then I am certain that you can mitigate this form of residual damage that herpes could have on your relationship.

The 'Oh Yeah' Syndrome

I also want to caution you not to throw herpes into the mix when you fight about something else altogether. It's easy to throw in the kitchen sink when you're having a fight. He blames her for losing the car keys and a few minutes later she's saying, "Oh yeah, well, you gave me herpes." I know it can be tempting to do this, but for the good of your relationship, avoid this temptation. It's a tactic you shouldn't use in general because it damages your relationship. If you can't counter with a comeback for your partner's last accusation, just walk away from the argument rather than starting to pull past hurts from your "Oh Yeah" drawer. Nobody wins when a fight has hit this stage, and the added damage such accusations make are not worth it. If you really care about the relationship, go for a walk around the block every time you and your partner are about to enter "Oh Yeah" mode.

Hanging On Because of Guilt

If either partner is hanging on to the relationship only out of guilt, that is not a wise idea. Guilt can keep two people together for a time, but eventually this type of glue will dry up and crack and the relationship will fall apart. A little guilt is okay. If you're extra nice to the other person because you feel bad for something you did to him or her, there's no harm in that. But if guilt is the only reason that one partner is remaining in the relationship, then that is a big problem.

At some point this partner is going to say to him or herself, "Why am I in this relationship? I don't love this person. Just because I gave them herpes doesn't mean that I have to be miserable for the rest of my life." Whenever this person reaches this conclusion, the guilty party will leave, and the person he or she gave herpes to will feel just as bad as if this breakup had occurred in the first place, plus they will have wasted all this time in a relationship that was destined to fail.

If Your Partner Didn't Give You Herpes

If you both have herpes, but other people gave each of you the disease, then the above situations are not ones that you're going to face. And yet both of you will still have to deal with the emotional effects of the disease. That should make you more sympathetic to each other, but again, that can happen only if your partner understands what has caused a particular emotional reaction. There are going to be times when you're going to be angry with each other that have nothing to do with herpes. If there's a particular act that has caused this anger, rather than fallout from herpes, then you're each entitled to defend yourselves (though you should never go overboard in a fight with a loved one). But if herpes is the cause, and you know it, then you each should cut the other some slack.

This would also be true if your partner had any disease or was enduring any other situation that was causing him or her a lot of stress. The main point I want to make here is that some emotional triggers are long-term—lifelong, in fact, in the case of herpes—and you need to develop a plan of action for dealing with them to prevent them from doing serious damage to your relationship. There's anger and then there's ANGER, and if you make sure that you can differentiate between the different types of anger, it will be much easier to learn to cope with such outbursts.

The Sorrow of Herpes

I've been using anger as an example more than sorrow, but the latter can be even tougher to deal with. First of all, it's not always as apparent. Anger often shows itself not in angry words or a frown, but through, say, a slammed door. Unless someone bursts into tears, or has the red eyes that show he or she has been crying recently, sadness can be overwhelming on the inside and not give a hint of the extent of the damage on the outside.

The other problem with sadness is that it can linger. Anger tends to dissipate after a while on its own. Your body probably couldn't stand all the chemical reactions that anger can cause— the flood of adrenaline, for example—for an extended period of time. But you can be sad for days on end, almost without a break. And if sadness lasts even longer, and becomes chronic, it can turn into depression.

While anger can disappear as quickly as it came, sadness usually doesn't come with an off switch. A wave of sorrow usually takes some time to disappear, so the partner of someone who is undergoing a bout of the blues can't expect to just give that person a hug, or tell them a joke, and hope for their sadness to evaporate. It takes more patience to deal with sadness, on the part of both partners.

Because of the lingering quality of sadness, it can have a more serious impact on a couple's sex life than anger. As you probably know, at least anecdotally, some couples will rush off to the bedroom right after a big fight. I guess it's all those chemical reactions I was just mentioning that set their sexual juices stirring. Sadness usually has just the opposite effect. Someone may be only a little bit sad but that can be enough to turn them off with regard to any desire for sex.

Because of the insidious nature of sadness, both partners will have to work fairly hard to overcome such an emotional reaction, whether it stems from herpes or from something else. You each have to take your time, lean on each other for comfort, and slowly pull up the sad person's spirits by showing your love for each other in myriad little ways. But the sad person must be willing to do his or her part, or the partner's efforts will be useless.

If this sadness becomes chronic and turns into what is called *clinical depression,* medical attention will be necessary. If you're not sure whether you or your partner is depressed rather than just sad, you should still go for a consultation. The earlier you get help, the sooner a solution can be found, so it's better to err on the side of caution than to avoid seeing a doctor just because you might be wrong and the case isn't severe enough for medical intervention.

Herpes Shouldn't Be a Crutch

At this point I want to add one caveat about all these emotional reactions you or your partner might get to herpes, and that is not to use them as a crutch. If one of you is constantly blaming herpes for every ill that befalls you, you will become like the boy who cried wolf. At some point your partner will no longer be able to be sympathetic, especially if it is clear that herpes is not to blame most of the time. You can reasonably ask your partner for sympathy, but if you do so unreasonably, then don't expect that you're going to get as much sympathy as you ask for, if any at all, after a time.

You also shouldn't use herpes as a way of avoiding sex. If every time your partner approaches you for sex you say, "Not tonight, I feel like an attack of herpes is coming," then that too won't be believable after a time. It's all right not to want sex, and while using a white lie once in a while is not something I'm against, using the same white lie over and over will be counterproductive.

When Only One Partner Has Herpes

Some of the advice I just gave applies to couples who are split: one with herpes and the other without. These couples must also learn to work out how to deal with the emotional baggage that herpes carries, and the advice I gave in the preceding section works for them as well. But such couples also face a different set of problems.

The one that can be the most difficult to navigate is the game plan required to keep the partner without herpes from getting it. When love first blooms, the partner without herpes may say that he or she doesn't really care. It's possible he or she is telling the truth at that moment in time and that if he or she came down with herpes, they wouldn't care, nor would they hold it against the other person. But it's difficult to predict the future, particularly when it comes to the reaction of someone who comes down with a severe case of painful herpes. Look at all the risky behavior that takes place despite the risks of getting AIDS, and how many risk-takers come to regret their past actions. People tend to be blasé about certain types of risks, and that is especially true when they're blinded by some strong emotion, be that either love or lust, or both. If they put themselves at risk often enough, at some point they're going to regret their actions. And that regret can extend to the very relationship that got them to this point in the first place.

So, my suggestion is to assume that it's important to try to keep your partner safe. Using valacyclovir is one way of doing that, though I would also caution you to use condoms and pay attention to any symptoms you might notice. Remember, the medications are effective, but they're not 100 percent effective. At least if you're both trying hard to prevent the transmission of herpes, if your partner does get herpes despite all your precautions, he or she will be less likely to put all the blame on you. If that forces you to play police-man, so be it. Since you're the one with herpes, you have to assume that responsibility. If you need to be the one to pull out the con-dom, even if you're not going to be the one to wear it, then shoul-der that duty without complaint. You just want to be as careful as possible so that you don't pass herpes on to your partner.

Adapting to herpes in this way will put a crimp in your sex life. There will be times when you won't be able to have sex. A male partner may resent the need to use a condom. And any nag-ging fear can put a damper on desire, even if you don't realize it. The key is to take stock of what is happening, assign the blame where it belongs, and then deal with it. Let me explain what I mean by this.

What I mean by taking stock is to communicate with each other about the status of your sex life. If there's something about your sex life that you think needs fixing, tell your partner about it. Whatever this problem is, it might not be possible to fix. For example, if keeping your partner safe from herpes requires the male to wear a condom, then there's nothing you can really do about it. But maybe you can compensate for this in other ways. Let's say that he would find it arousing if she would do a striptease for him but she feels silly doing that. By stripping for him, though, she will increase his level of arousal, which will compensate, to some extent, for his having to wear a condom. So even if she feels silly, she should strip for him once in a while. Now you should never do anything under pressure that really bothers you. For example, if he wants anal sex and she hates the idea, then she has the right to say no. But if it's something that you don't love but also don't find too distasteful, then to make up for the complication of having herpes, and to show your love for your partner, it would appropriate to go ahead and grant this type of request, at least from time to time.

To help you assign the blame for these types of issues, you almost have to look at herpes as a third party to your relationship. You have to say to yourself, "It's not my partner's fault; it's the fault of herpes." If it helps you, I suggest getting a rubber ball and calling it herpes. Then when you get really mad at the disease, you can throw the ball against the wall or out of the room, or even out of the house. The disease won't actually leave with that ball, but some of the frustrations may disappear for a while.

So dealing with these issues means identifying them, talking about them, and then finding creative ways to soften their edges. The biggest mistake you can make is to ignore them, because then they have a chance to silently grow in importance and get so big that handling them will be very difficult, if not impossible.

Actually, going the extra mile to please your partner is a good idea whether you are dealing with herpes or not. It can only strengthen the relationship, as long as both halves of the couple go out of their way for each other and it's not always a one-way street, which will end up having a negative effect.

What if, despite all your precautions, your partner does get herpes? Does it spell the end of your relationship? Hopefully not. Even if your partner has a bad initial reaction and ends up blaming you, despite having vowed over and over again not to, you have to understand what your partner is going through. It's difficult to accept blame for your own stupidity. It's easier to blame someone else, even if you know it's not their fault. So my advice is to cut them some slack for a while. You remember how traumatic it was for you when you first got herpes, and so you need to let them adjust to having undergone this significant change in their health status. If they act as if they're angry with you, even if they say they aren't, let it slide off your back for a while. Don't react to their anger by getting angry yourself. Stop yourself from saying "I told you so," no matter how great the temptation. If you feel you can't stifle angry words, then say them to yourself in a mirror. Or to your partner while they're sleeping. Or mouth the words to their back. Or write them a letter that you never send. Sometimes it is tough, maybe impossible, to keep silent, but that doesn't mean the other person has to hear you. If you really feel that you have to say angry words, do it in a way that will do the least harm to your relationship.

The emotional reaction of a partner who gets herpes could end up being very severe. They may not be able to contain their anger. Or they may become very depressed. Their level of desire might drop to zero and they won't want to have sex anymore, which would not be an entirely surprising reaction given that sex was the cause of getting the disease. Part of a severe reaction could be a shutdown in communications. If this person suddenly clams up, making repairs is going to be an impossible process. So if you do encounter an extreme reaction, don't try to handle it all by yourselves. At that point, go for professional counseling.

It might be tempting to say you know the cause of the reaction, herpes, and so you don't need any type of therapy. But not all types of therapists need to discover the root of the problem in order to help the person. Sometimes just getting a third party involved who can act as a mediator is what is required. If the partners aren't telling each other what they're really thinking, but will open up to this third party, then the therapist serves a very important purpose. And while partners may ignore each other's suggestions, they may give more credence to the words of a professional, even if the advice is quite obvious and they could have thought of it themselves. It can also be helpful to know that someone is looking over your shoulder. You might be less likely to start a fight if you know that it will be the subject of your next session.

I would advise a couple going through difficulties not to wait to seek professional help. The longer you're at each other's throats, or a depressed person is moping around, the harder it will be to make the needed repairs. It's much like a plumbing problem. If you don't fix a leak while it's little, it's likely to get bigger, and so more damaging, and be much harder, and more expensive, to repair. So once you feel that the situation is not one that you can handle alone, go for help.

Your first step needn't be someone who charges you by the hour. Perhaps you have a religious leader whom you like and trust who could act as an intermediary. Or if you go to a local hospital, there may be a social worker who could be of assistance. I might suggest going to a support group, but if one of you has already gone to the one in your area, I could see a potential problem if the partner who then gets herpes perceives this group as friends of their partner and not as a neutral body that could give impartial advice or counseling. It's an issue you could bring up with the group leader and see if there might be a way of addressing it. This will certainly depend on the group leader and how he or she feels about handling such a situation. Just remember, group leaders may be very good at helping people who need assistance in coping with herpes, but that doesn't make them experts at couples therapy. If the relationship is really on rocky ground, then a professional therapist will be required.

Chapter Highlights

1. Just because both partners have herpes doesn't mean that issues won't arise in their relationship that are caused by herpes.
2. Emotional outbursts handled as a team will do the least harm to your relationship.
3. Be creative in finding ways of handling this third party in your relationship, herpes.
4. If the problem requires professional counseling, don't delay in getting the help you need.

8

Support Groups

Shannon—I am so grateful for the support groups, chat rooms, and dating sites on the Internet for people who have herpes. It took me seven years of feeling like I was alone with this disease until I got access to the Internet and started finding the other people who have it. It feels good to be truly understood by someone who's been there. I've met a lot of good friends in the support groups and chat rooms and have met a few people from the dating sites. I've spent many hours in the herpes chat room. I've listened to many different stories, tried to help out the newcomers and give the best possible advice I could, and I've made a lot of friends along the way.

I've heard that some people have been known to show up at a herpes support group meeting only hours after they've received their diagnosis, while someone like Shannon took seven years. I've been telling people that this book is supposed to be like a support group, especially for those who have been unable to connect with one, but as good as this book might be, for someone going through the trauma of having herpes, there is no substitute to actually listening to and talking with real people who have herpes and have undergone a similar ordeal.

> **Anna**—I debated over whether I should tell my family and decided against it. I have been a very private person all my life, and I couldn't see that changing. The support groups I have found have changed my perspective on sharing somewhat, and I have been making attempts at opening up more.

When you were a child and you skinned your knee, the first person you ran to was Mom. She could give you comfort that no one else could, though Dad and grandparents were a close second. As you grew older, and your problems went from scrapes to heartaches, it was perhaps a sibling that you felt most comfortable opening up to. We humans need to talk things out and family members are often the ones we turn to because after all, we've known them all our lives. But when it comes to a subject like herpes, a family member might not always be appropriate. Any time sex is the subject matter, it becomes more difficult to communicate honestly with a family member. Families tend to be the bodies that try to hold you back when it comes to sex, so if you catch a sexually transmitted disease, you're going to be worried that you're more likely to get a scolding than comfort, even if that's not true. But since everyone in the support group has herpes too, it's one place where you can be sure you and your disease will be welcomed with open arms.

> **Slacapra**—When I was first diagnosed with herpes, I was told by my physician that as long as I used condoms, I didn't have to tell anyone I had herpes. Eight years later when I finally joined a support group I learned so much more about the disease and I was horrified. I, like so many others before and after me, had been given inappropriate direction by someone I felt that I

should be able to trust, my physician! I quickly integrated into the small group and within months of finding the group had acquired enough basic information about the virus to fulfill the testing provided by ASHA (American Social Health Association) and keep the help group from ending due to lack of a cofacilitator.

I work with doctors, have many doctors as friends, and have a great deal of respect for them. But I also know that many doctors get somewhat tongue-tied when the subject matter has to do with sexual functioning. And if they're embarrassed, then the information they pass on to patients isn't always complete. On the other hand, sometimes a little knowledge can be a dangerous thing. If a layperson gives you medical advice, they might leave out some important facts or give you information that is erroneous. But if instead of one person telling you something you hear it in front of a group, many of whose members are quite knowledgeable, then that changes matters. If one person says something that is wrong, chances are that several others will correct him. And if nothing else, you'll at least come away with the right questions to ask a physician.

Fred—I'm not a joiner. The idea of going to a support group was not something I thought I'd ever do. But I needed to talk to somebody and at that point I was too ashamed to tell any of my friends or family. The night of the meeting, I walked past the door a couple of times, not knowing if I could actually go through with it. It was like a movie. I literally took a deep breath before pushing the door open.

The hardest part about going to a support group is that very first step of crossing the threshold. This may be difficult for people without herpes to understand, but if your ego has been crushed by this disease, the last thing you want to do is announce to a group of people that you have herpes. Rationally you may know that they all have herpes, but because they're already part of this group, emotionally this knowledge doesn't really help.

What you have to tell yourself is that an experience like this one is similar to having to go to the dentist when you have a toothache. Of course it's not a pleasant thought, but after you've sat in the dentist's chair, you're going to feel relief from the pain you're suffering. And after you've attended a support group meeting, you're going to feel relief from the psychic pain that herpes has inflicted on you. So it's important that you make the effort no matter how much you dread it.

> **Ruth**—Even though I love my boyfriend and know he loves me I still had to battle the feelings that society labels you with: worthlessness, feelings of being dirty, being used, and being a slut. Bearing in mind that my boyfriend was only the second guy I've ever slept with, most of these feelings were unjustified, but it doesn't stop you feeling them.

Visiting a support group is a way of cleansing your psyche of its insecurities. Imagine getting dressed in the morning, heading out for the day, and discovering that you have a rather large stain somewhere on your clothes. Most people won't notice it. The few who do won't really care. But you feel contaminated. You can't wait to get back home and rip off that stained article of clothing. We all feel that way when this happens to us. And that's the way you feel when you have herpes, only there are no visible signs of it, and there's nothing you can rip off at the end of the day. But what you can do is learn to accept yourself, and that's where support groups come in.

> **Amanda**—When I decided that I needed the help of a support group, I called and was just in time for an upcoming meeting.

It was so great. The people were so nice to me. There were thirty people there, all with herpes. Afterward we went out for pizza, which we ended up doing every Thursday night, talking until midnight. Having a group of friends with herpes really helped me.

Amanda is an outgoing type of person, and wound up becoming the head of the New York support group. But everyone needs at least one friend they can pour their heart out to. Since it's so hard to talk about herpes to people who don't have it, finding a group of people who do can be such a blessing. You know they're not going to be judgmental about your having herpes since they all have it. And you also know you can say anything to them because they're not going to look at you strangely. At some point you may not need the support group anymore, and that's fine, but some of these people will become friends beyond the realm of herpes, and any time you can add to your list of friends, that's a wonderful opportunity as well.

Amy—I only had herpes for three weeks when I went to my first Indy Gathering. Three hundred people, all with herpes. It was so moving that I couldn't keep from crying. I had been scared to death but when I saw three hundred people like me, I wanted to live. There was such a feeling of fellowship. There were picnics, dances. People met mentors for life. It's a touching and priceless environment. A true sense of community.

Most support group meetings are on the small side, but you can imagine what it must be like to have hundreds of people gathered together. If a room full of people can make you feel more normal, having a huge crowd can help you strip away all the guilt and shame you've been feeling. It's one thing to read that millions of people have herpes; it's another to actually see a crowd of people giving living proof to that statistic.

Ron—Even though I cannot change the world of people who have H, I can make a difference. I truly believe the Lord has given me this "gift" to help others. After joining many of these social groups, I have been able to do that. Many members are "newbies," and don't know how to deal with H. And besides, I wouldn't have met so many wonderful people across the nation whom I consider family. These national events are like a family reunion!!!

I mentioned the difficulties of telling your family, and in some cases, having herpes can mean losing touch with your family—if not actually, then emotionally, because if you are carrying around a secret that you don't feel comfortable revealing to them, the close feelings you once had for them will be blocked by this wall. But you need people with whom you feel close, and support groups can provide you with a new family.

And whether you consider the people in a support group your family or just friends, the fact that once you've reestablished your emotional balance with regard to herpes and your life you can then help others can be very important. Making something positive out of something negative will make it so much easier to deal with.

Alan—I visited a help group that was a two-hour trip away. Became interested and started a help group in my local area. I started it six years ago and now the others have faded away and ours is the only one left. The group leaders are all volunteers and after a while they get tired and wear out.

Part of being a family is that you are not a guest. When it's time for the family to eat, all the members pitch in and help, or at least they ought to. If you go to a group meeting, keep in mind that the leader is not being paid to devote so much time to helping others but is volunteering him or herself. They get a lot back, which is why they continue, but it can be of immense psychological help if they feel that other members of the group are acting like family members and actively supporting the group with both time and effort. If you're getting a lot from a group you're in, don't forget to give something back.

> **Mark**—The power of a self-help group can be seen by the number of people who drop out. After a few weeks they've achieved what they wanted and can go back to their lives. Some come back, particularly if they're about to start a new relationship. They may want to try out the conversation they're going to have with this new person by doing role play.

In addition to the support of these groups, they can also be testing grounds. It's one thing to have a conversation with your mirror, another to have it with a live person who can respond. That's especially true if this other person has undergone this type of conversation in real life and can bring to it his or her experiences, as can, of course, the other people in the room. And once you have a number of people tell you that you're ready for The Talk, that will also raise your level of self-confidence, making it even more likely that you'll be successful.

> **Mary**—Don't tell anyone you're not sleeping with that you have it, unless you're in an anonymous support group. It's not a good idea because people who don't have it may not understand.

Mary told a girlfriend who then told the man she was interested in to steal him away from her. Not every friend is going to try something like that, but you never know. I'm always in favor of being extra careful about private matters. You can certainly tell a therapist anything you want because it will never leave the room, but when it comes to others, you never know. If you're in a support group where you can remain anonymous, though, you can use such a group to talk out your problems without the risk of any secrets getting into the wrong hands.

> **Betsy**—A year ago I found an online support group that I liked. It helps me to keep current on new advances in genital herpes and it lets me help newly diagnosed people cope with having herpes. There is so much misinformation out there. Most doctors don't seem to understand enough to teach their patients. There are so many questions people are afraid to ask their doctors about herpes and sex. The online group gives them an anonymous place to ask them where they don't have to look anyone in the eye while doing so.

> **Stephanie**—I went online in search of information and support, and found both. They were a lifesaver. The moderator, in particular, was very knowledgeable, and explained to me that in fact, the human body takes twelve to sixteen weeks to manufacture antibodies to the virus—therefore, if you have a positive culture on a lesion, and a negative blood test, you know that you were having a "primary outbreak" and had contracted the virus within the past sixteen weeks. Well, I hadn't been with anyone else for much longer than that, so I had my answer, but I was appalled that the midwife had not known that. I then went to my internist for the blood test (Western blot, the gold standard), and found out that she, too, did not know about the antibody issue.

While online support groups cannot match a group of live people for giving you emotional support, they're a wonderful place to start; as far as getting pure information, they can be as good as a real-world support group. But if you surf the Web, then you also know that there are other sites that offer misinformation. So it's important that you're careful when searching. Included in the back of this book is an appendix of various sites that have good information. If you start from this, you can't go wrong. And if you find other information that you're not sure about, then check it on one of these sites for accuracy.

By the way, I'm constantly being offered endorsement deals for some vitamin product or other that purports to improve your sexual appetite. I turn these down as a matter of course. And I know that there are also so-called natural remedies for herpes. Such products may have a positive effect, particularly if you believe in them, but in my opinion, they possess no true curative powers, but rather, may work via the placebo effect.

Online Support Groups

While I'm giving you warnings, I have to also pass on a warning about online support groups. While most of the people who go on them to chat or meet other people are legitimate, some are only "trawling," that is to say looking for someone with whom to make a connection while hiding their true identity. In other words, they may say that they have herpes, but they may not. And all the other information they give you about themselves may also be false. This can happen on any site where chatting goes on, but because people with herpes are somewhat more vulnerable than the norm, it does present a bigger danger.

If you've been afraid of dating because of having to reveal that you have herpes, and someone on one of these sites acts very sympathetically to you, it may give you new hope. In that case, you might be more likely to want to actually meet this person, and if this person is not who or what they say they are, then who knows who they really are and what dangers they may pose? I don't want to be extra negative, especially to a group of people who do have special needs because of having herpes, but I would be remiss in not pointing out the dangers. Remember, many of you reading this book got herpes from someone who knew they had it but failed to tell you about it. That's a very vivid example of how nasty some human beings can be. So having been burned once, don't make the same mistake again.

Chapter Highlights

1. It may be very hard to get up the courage to go to a support group, but the end result will be well worth it.
2. Support groups can act like a family without making you feel guilty.
3. Online support groups have much to offer but also present dangers.

9
Talking to Your Kids about Herpes

There are some topics that parents really enjoy talking to their kids about—for example, telling them about the music they listened to or television shows they watched when they were growing up. Other topics are a bit more uncomfortable. Perhaps you used drugs when you were younger (or maybe still do) but you don't want your children imitating you. Then you have to decide whether you want to admit to any drug usage on your side or just give them an antidrug message, leaving your personal information aside. Talking to your kids about herpes falls somewhere in between these two ends of the spectrum, depending on how you got it.

> **Betsy**—When they are a bit older I will tell my children I have genital herpes and explain it to them. I just hope my bad luck in getting herpes will help them to be more aware of STDs in general so they take the effort to protect themselves against STDs when they are sexually active.

Telling Your Story

As we've seen in this book, some people with herpes got it because they were promiscuous, but most weren't. One could say that for the latter group it was mostly a case of bad luck, but with herpes being so widespread, the odds of getting it aren't all that low. But if you want to keep your kids from getting herpes, or any STD, then you do have to make sure they understand how easy it is for it to happen to them. And, of course, there's no better way of convincing them of that than by letting them know that one, or both, of their parents have an STD.

> **Stephanie**—I've had discussions about sex with my son for quite some time, but the birth control one is next. A discussion of STDs will be part of that. Again, calm and direct is the way to go. I don't honestly know if I'll tell him yet that I have HSV. Probably not for a few years, but I could change my mind.

Knowing that a parent caught an STD would certainly help get the message about the dangers of STDs across to a child. But telling your child that you have herpes could also be quite embarrassing, at least to many people. If you do tell your children that you have herpes, it will place all your discussions about sex on a more honest plane. It will probably make you more of an "askable parent," which is important because if your children don't feel that they can turn to you for information about sex, then they'll get it somewhere else, which would mean that it could be wrong, and certainly won't have the moral message that you would want to convey along with it. But telling them will also open up a basketful of questions, starting off with "How did you get it?" That may then lead to a whole discussion of your past sex life, which you might not want to reveal to them.

Because of these issues, you have to plan ahead for any such discussion. If you keep putting off how you intend to deal with this, your child may come home from school with some questions that will force the issue into the open and then you might have to figure out what to say on the fly, which could be troublesome. Remember, there's no need to tell your child that you have an STD. If it would make you uncomfortable, you have my permission to keep this fact about your life a secret. Since you do know your story quite well, you could always use it as an example, but say it's something you know about a friend and you can't tell them who that friend is. Using a white lie like this will lessen the impact of the lesson, but it will also save both of you from some embarrassment, and that may be a worthwhile payoff. But just don't put off having this discussion for too long or the subject of herpes, or some other STD, may come up because your child has caught it.

Keeping Children Safe

Julie—I got type 1 herpes from my husband from oral sex and it turned into a very severe case of genital herpes. I do not let my children use the same towels I have used.

Of course, there may be aspects of having herpes that you don't want to hide from your kids because you don't want them to catch it from you. To the extent that they need to know that you have an illness of some sort that you don't want them to catch, you can tell a child of any age that they must be careful. (You can't catch herpes from a towel, but if you have a cold sore on your mouth, then it would be catching if they kissed you on the mouth, for example.) You don't necessarily have to tell them how you got the disease if you feel they're too young to have to deal with that side of herpes. You only have to give them the information you feel they need to know to avoid catching it from you.

Making Use of the Opportunity

Of course, at the time you are telling them about herpes 1 and cold sores, you could also let them know about genital herpes. They may squirm a bit when you switch the subject, but since it's a very good way of introducing this type of discussion, don't let them squeeze out of it.

This might also be a good time to check out what your kids are being taught in school. Ask them if they have been told about STDs in any sex-ed classes and try to find out how much of the information they were given stuck. If a roomful of kids are embarrassed, chances are they won't be paying very close attention. If they're supposed to know about STDs and from your questioning you see that your child doesn't even know the basics, then you know that you have to go into more depth on this subject matter. It doesn't have to be during this particular discussion. In fact, you may want to bone up on the subject of the other STDs before you talk to your child. But, again, don't put it off indefinitely or by the time you have the discussion, it might be too late.

I would strongly advise you get some pamphlets on the various STDs that you could show them. (Or you can print out some material from the Web.) First of all, it's a lot of information to absorb, even for you. And the pamphlets will have diagrams and graphs that will make it easier to show your child. You can give them the pamphlets so they can look at them on their own. They might be embarrassed while you're talking to them, and that will make it harder for them to listen to what you are saying. But if you've made them at least pay attention to the dangers, then they can look at the specifics later on.

Teens Think They Know It All

Anna—One thing that struck me and has helped me were two realizations: (1) that I was not alone, and (2) that I was grateful I was in my mid-thirties and not high school or college-aged. Having experienced emotional and physical trauma at a younger age, I know that I am now better equipped to handle this.

Teens think that they're all grown up and know all they need to know about everything, but we adults know differently. That many teens are almost fearless is a good thing, because they have a world to conquer and you don't want them starting out in it being afraid of their shadow. On the other hand, there are real dangers out there from which you want to protect them, and finding the middle ground can be difficult.

When I give a lecture, I don't allow anyone under eighteen to attend. That's because the message I give to adults, which is that whatever two consenting adults want to do is okay by me, is not appropriate for teens. On the other hand, when I address an audience of teens, I don't allow a single adult to sit in the room. That's because I know that the teens won't open up to me the way they will if it's just them and me. (Their teachers don't always like it, but I insist and they always back down.)

But while I can develop a certain rapport with an audience of teens for a limited amount of time, you as a parent must maintain that role throughout the year. In order to help them resist peer pressure, which is very strong in the teen years, they need to know that Mom or Dad would punish them if they got caught doing this or that. So how do you remain an askable parent while being an authority figure? One way is by maintaining everyone's privacy. By speaking in abstract terms, rather than personal ones, you can talk about birth control without condoning sexual activity on their part. But privacy is a two-way street, and you need to maintain your privacy too. That's why, as I said earlier, you don't necessarily have to tell your children that you have herpes.

Now I know that there are many herpes "activists" who feel that one of the worst parts about getting herpes is the emotional pain, which comes mostly because people think of herpes as a horrible sexually transmitted disease, and that the way to get around that is to be as open as possible when it comes to discussing herpes. Those people are going to want to tell their children everything there is to know about herpes, including the fact that they have it. But while it's okay for an adult to be open, it's another thing for a teen. Teens haven't figured it all out yet (not that we adults have either) and they need more privacy than adults, more space in which to grow. And they don't want to know about their parents' sex lives because they're still sorting out their own. So while I understand the urge to reveal all to your children, I continue to urge caution in that respect.

If you're on the fence about this question, one way of dealing with it is rather than offering to tell your children that you have herpes, to wait until they ask about it. It might take them a while to put two and two together and hopefully when the question does come up, they'll be old enough to understand the answers better. But if because of herpes your teen does learn that you were having sex before you were married, don't be surprised to have that set of circumstances thrown back at you someday. At some point you may want to convince a child not to go too far with a boyfriend or girlfriend and they're going to say, "You did it, so why can't I?" It might be tempting at that time to retort with "I got herpes because of it," but I don't think that will be effective. As I've said before, scare tactics usually don't work. Your child is likely to skip over that line of reasoning, saying that they'll take precautions to be safe, and instead concentrate on the fact that premarital sex is okay.

On the other hand, if you know that your child is sexually active, then you may, if you want, use the fact that you have herpes to try to convince them to follow safer sex practices. Make sure that condoms are available and let them know all that you've found out about testing for STDs.

Talk to Your Kids

Deanne—I was pregnant and my ex-husband talked me into having unprotected sex. Since I couldn't get pregnant *again,* I didn't think we needed to use a condom, and so he ended up giving me herpes, and as a result I lost the baby. I don't want the death of my child to be in vain. My child would now be nineteen, in the prime of his or her life, so if this is a way I can help the community understand the psychology behind the disease, and its implications, I will do what it takes.

But, again, don't let this issue of whether or not to tell your children that you have herpes or any other STD get in the way of telling them about this and all STDs. What Deanne's ex-husband did to her was terrible and there was nothing she could do to prevent it, but that doesn't mean that many other people can't protect themselves, as long as they know how. So your duty as a parent is above all to inform your children of the dangers. You shouldn't scare them, but you must make sure that this information sinks in. Their schools are supposed to be doing this, but the end result may not always be that comprehensible to your child, as many teachers of sex education are not properly prepared, and so either don't have the right information or haven't enough training to overcome their own embarrassment. So this is one area in which you have to reinforce their education. At the very least, get them some material—pamphlets, books, and so on—that you can give them to read. They are curious about anything having to do with sex and they probably will read this information. So if you can find information that provides them with the facts and also agrees with your moral values, then you'll have accomplished much of the goal, even if you don't do much talking yourself.

Chapter Highlights

1. It's important that you make sure your children know about STDs.
2. You don't have to tell them that you have herpes.
3. When talking to teens, allow them to maintain their privacy.

10
Herpes and Seniors

While many young people assume that older adults don't have a sex life, it's absolutely not true. Certainly there are changes that occur with aging that will alter the sex lives of both men and women, but we humans can go on having sex until we're in our nineties, and maybe even beyond. And what too many older adults fail to realize is that if one is sexually active, it is quite possible to catch a sexually transmitted disease such as herpes.

One of the changes that older women go through that may lead to getting an STD is menopause. Up until this point in their lives, women have to worry about preventing an unintended pregnancy. That tends to make them extra careful and to take every precaution when having sex. Then they go through menopause and that fear evaporates. They no longer have to think about using some form of contraception, including condoms. If they're with a husband and he's remained monogamous, then there's no need to worry about STDs. But if they're single or if their husband has strayed, then menopause or not, they are as vulnerable to getting an STD as younger women.

Sonya—I believed that I had everything all figured out. My life was on a great track: my daughters grown and independent, my grandson healthy and beautiful, and my career on track.

I wanted to experiment with the free life. I had been married for eleven years and with a man after my divorce for another eight, always faithfully. On my own after those years and being so "good," I wanted to experiment!

I was getting dressed for work and the phone rang.

"Is Amy there?"

"No, I am sorry, you have the wrong number."

I was about to hang up and he said: "Wait! Are you sure you were not online last night talking to me?"

I laughed. Great line!

"Nope," I said. "It is not me."

"Listen, you have a great voice. Do you think we could meet for coffee?"

My mind reeled. A stranger, just the excitement that I was looking for. All those people that I know who spent their twenties experimenting and having fun while I raised kids and stayed steady.

"Yes, I would love to."

When I went to meet him at 7-Eleven, I had this gnawing feeling inside me that I should just go home—he seemed shifty. But I suppressed my instincts and invited him back to my apartment.

He spent the weekend with me and we made love without a condom, unprotected. He had a cold that he was "getting over." He left on Sunday and I never heard from him again.

Tuesday morning, I broke out. It was awful. It was painful and it lasted for twelve weeks. I went to the Public Health Department, because I was ashamed to go to my doctor.

An old woman, my age, getting diseased for a fling after all these years. A grandmother, for heaven's sake. I cried for days.

If Sonya had been younger, she never would have had unprotected sex because she would have been afraid of getting pregnant. But with that fear gone, it didn't occur to her to protect herself from herpes.

Of course, a younger woman might not have had this fling to begin with. Many older women become prey to men like this because it is more difficult for them to find a partner. As people get older, there are fewer and fewer available men and the women who are left just can't be as choosy, especially as the men their age that are around are mostly married. So when the opportunity to feel desirable comes along, they're more likely to grab it, especially as they feel the risks aren't as great since they can't become pregnant. But as Sonya learned, that can be a dangerous trap.

This imbalance in the sexes can have the opposite effect for men. An older man, who perhaps had problems finding women to go to bed with when he was younger, might suddenly find a line of women banging on his door. He may have been married for years and become a widower, and the availability of all these women makes him decide that the time to sow his wild oats is at the end of his life, assuming he didn't also do so earlier on. And with there being no need of using a condom to prevent pregnancy, he's not likely to carry any on his forays into these various bedrooms. But as a result, even if he didn't have herpes or some other disease when he started, the odds increase with each new conquest that he will catch something, and then spread it to the other women he beds.

To some extent the prevalence of STDs among older adults is less, so if everyone stays within a tight circle, such as a retirement community where there currently is no one with an STD, it may be possible for lots of people to have sex with each other without spreading any diseases. (I'm not saying here that every community of older people resembles some Roman orgy, but if there are enough single adults living in close proximity, you can be sure that at least some of them are having sex.) But you can't count on that. All it takes is one infected person to join this group and very quickly an entire community can get herpes, or some other STD.

The obvious answer is for older adults who have sex with people with whom they don't have a relationship to use condoms. But the dynamics I've been mentioning can make it difficult. If an older woman hasn't had sex in a while and along comes a suitor who refuses to use a condom, what is she to do? It's easy to say that she should just walk away from the situation, but I know how difficult it can be. What can make it even more difficult is that if this woman turns the man down, her next-door neighbor may take him in. If it turns out that he doesn't have any diseases, her neighbor may have made a catch that won't come along in the near future, if ever again. That can be a very strong incentive not to turn this man down.

The answer to this problem is that older adults need to be more open about talking about herpes and other STDs. There has to be an awareness within each such community that STDs are out there and pose a threat. In other words, there has to be some peer pressure created so that as many women as possible will insist on using safer sex practices so that a gentleman with a disease has less of a chance of infecting everyone he comes into contact with. (This would also apply to a woman with a disease who had sex with lots of men, but the entire premise of this particular issue is based around the statistical fact that as we humans age, there are many more single women around than single men, so it is the single older men who are more likely to have multiple partners.)

One of the arguments that an older man may use against using condoms is that because he is older he has a harder time obtaining and maintaining an erection, and that a condom will make it impossible for him to do so. It is true that an older man might need more stimulation to get an erection, and that he can lose it more easily, though with the new drugs against erectile difficulties, that is not necessarily true (though older men with heart conditions cannot use Viagra or its new counterparts). The alternative to condom use, then, is for the man to get tested. If he can prove that he is disease-free, then a potential partner needn't worry about catching any diseases. Of course, testing for herpes can be difficult, and a false negative is possible if someone got herpes only recently. Given the realities of the situation, that older single women do have a hard time finding sexual partners, I suppose some risks are unavoidable. But such women can't ignore the risks altogether and should do all they can to protect themselves. So if condoms are not a possible solution (and as we know, they don't provide complete protection against herpes either), then testing must be part of the overall answer to keeping this segment of the population safe from herpes and other STDs.

Let me say one thing about the silver-lining effect here. While two young people can hop into the sack and quickly achieve sexual satisfaction, older people need more time and more intimacy. An older man probably won't have what is called a *psychogenic erection,* which is an erection that arises of its own, caused by, say, looking at an erotic photograph. Older men need physical stimulation to get an erection. And older women probably require the use of a lubricant and they, too, may need more stimulation to have an orgasm than they did when they were younger. So two older adults really should communicate before and during sex so that they can help each other get the most out of having sex together. By their having The Talk, which as we've seen helps to break down many of the communication barriers, it should also be easier for them to talk about their sexual needs.

Chapter Highlights

1. Older people are not immune to STDs.
2. If condom usage isn't possible, then testing should be insisted on.
3. Talking openly about sexual matters can be even more important to older people.

11
Herpes and Gays

For the most part, it doesn't make much of a difference whether you are gay or straight when it comes to herpes. Unlike AIDS, which once was primarily a disease passed on by homosexuals, herpes has always affected people of all sexual preferences equally. But there are some issues with regard to the gay population and herpes that need to be addressed.

The first one is that having herpes may increase the odds of getting HIV. In the countries in Africa where HIV is making the most serious inroads, herpes runs rampant. Though it hasn't been 100 percent proven, the evidence strongly suggests that someone who has herpes is more susceptible to getting HIV. Herpes lesions are like doorways through which the virus that causes AIDS can easily pass if someone is having unprotected sex. Though HIV is definitely a growing problem among heterosexuals, in this country it remains a bigger problem in the gay community, and so spreading the news about the potential effects of herpes on HIV is very important. Anyone with herpes has to realize that they are probably more open to getting HIV and so they should be even more cautious than ever—though nobody, gay or straight, should practice unsafe sex.

Dangerous Behavior

Larry—Would I tell everyone I was remotely interested in sex with that I had herpes? Would I stay celibate until I had met the "right one" and told him all about it, and had been accepted? I felt that not revealing it in any circumstance would be deeply unethical and thus agonized for months. I slowly came to a kind of uneasy moral compromise. If I wanted to play with the rough-and-ready guys who go to sex clubs I would, and would not feel the need to tell, but anyone I met and began a dating or communicative friendship with would need to know if I felt we might be heading toward intimacy. So I had some rough-and-ready casual sex, and also dated a few men. I spoke to a few other gay men about herpes, and it seems that "Don't ask, don't tell" is the rule with STDs these days. I also got the impression from a few comments that HIV/AIDS is somehow "cool" because it lends itself to an air of noble sociopolitical suffering, but herpes is nothing more than "icky" and quite unmentionable.

Am I shocked by what Larry had to say? In some sense, yes, but I'm not entirely surprised. I keep up with the news of the gay community and so I know that many gays, especially the younger ones who haven't witnessed all their friends dying from AIDS, do not always practice safer sex. There is this feeling that because of the so-called cocktails of medicine against AIDS, it no longer is a disease to be feared.

It's wonderful that there is something that people with AIDS can do to extend their lives, but not only are these drugs very expensive, and not always covered by insurance, but their effects also don't last forever. At best they delay the progression of HIV. But many with HIV infection are going to have their life cut short at some point in the future, unless new drugs are soon developed. And while these drugs can be effective, their side effects are not always pleasant. So to put it bluntly, HIV is not "cool" but is a deadly infection that should be avoided like—well, like the plague. Sadly too many gay people, judging by their actions, are ignoring this warning. And the type of behavior that can lead someone to get AIDS will also lead to getting all sorts of other STDs, including herpes, which means that with so many more people infected with HSV than HIV, herpes is certainly having a field day within the gay community. I suppose it should go without saying, but since it doesn't, I feel the necessity of putting my two cents in by saying that all gays should develop a relationship, and, until they do, not engage in any risky behavior. They must remember that any time there is an exchange of bodily fluids, there is a risk for disease to be transmitted. It may be ironic that a group of people who cannot cause an unintended pregnancy must take even more precautions than those who can, but that's just the way it is.

Prejudice Is Based on Myths

Martha—I'm more closeted about having herpes than being a lesbian. After all, no one can catch being a lesbian.

Though Martha's right, technically, I'm not sure that some of the prejudice aimed at gays doesn't come from some inner fear that some straight people have that they might become gay if they associate with gay people. It's certainly not true, unless they've been hiding their true sexual identity from the world, and themselves.

And, of course, there are many people who are afraid of catching herpes, or any STD, from towels or toilet seats, and those are also myths. But just because something is not true doesn't necessarily reduce its power. If people want to believe that something is true even though it's not, it's hard to dissuade them. It's these false truths that are the basis for most prejudice in the world. And as we saw in Larry's comments, some people will hold on to these false truths, such as the one that says it's cool to have AIDS, no matter how much evidence to the contrary is presented to them.

While it's a good thing to keep an open mind, I'm also a strong believer in making up my mind only when I have solid facts. For example, there are often "studies" reported in the press. When one of these studies has to do with sex, the media often call on me for my opinion. But I won't give an opinion unless I can see the full study ahead of time. The reason for this is that many of these so-called studies are merely polls that are not scientific. In other words, they don't mean a thing. But people will act on such a study even though it may not be true. For example, there have been all sorts of propositions put out as to why people are gay, but not one of these has been scientifically proven. The only thing we know for sure is that there are people who can become aroused only by having sex with someone of their own sex, rather than with the opposite one. You can't talk about whose fault it is or whether or not their behavior can be changed because there is no hard evidence relating to these concepts. You just have to accept them the way they are, just the way right-handed people accept left-handed people. In the not so distant past, lefties were forced to write with their right hand. That was wrong, and it would be wrong to try to force gays to have sex with the opposite sex. But that doesn't give gays free rein to have unsafe sex, any more than heterosexuals should. No one has the right to pass on an STD, whether it be herpes or HIV or any other one. Of course, it may happen by accident. With 90 percent of those with herpes not knowing it, that's definitely a possibility. But if you do know that you have an STD, then you must do everything in your power to prevent passing it on, no matter what your sexual orientation.

Support Groups Are Mostly Straight

Martha—When I was first diagnosed with herpes, back in the early '80s, I was the only lesbian in the support group I went to in New York. It was hard for a lesbian to relate to the group. All the talk was about condoms, which didn't help me, and there wasn't a word mentioned about dental dams.

I once taught a class at Brooklyn College in human sexuality that was only for the handicapped. They were a wonderful group of students but I vowed never to teach such a course again. My reason? I thought that the lessons these students could provide healthy students, and vice versa, were too important to isolate these individuals. From that experience, although I recognize that it may pose some difficulties for a gay person to join a support group that is mostly heterosexual, I believe, strongly, that it shouldn't stop them. You may be told some information that isn't appropriate, like a lesbian hearing about condom usage, but overall I think the experience would be very worthwhile. As we've seen throughout this book, the basic problems people encounter with herpes are human issues, and so apply to anyone faced with the guilt and shame that herpes can bring on an individual.

Martha—I've become a safe sex queen. Safe sex isn't about the technical apparatus but whether a person is really committed to working hard to do the right thing. This is particularly difficult to do if you're in an altered state. That's why you should try to negotiate that stuff during dinner before your brain chemistry shifts. I once called the CDC to ask about their research on using saran wrap instead of a dental dam and they didn't have any. I only learned about this as an alternative because it was being talked about. When I was first using it all I could do was hope for the best. Then I heard not to use the microwavable stuff because it wasn't impermeable. I've used dental dams. Actually they're much improved. I order them from Eve's Garden, which sells cute ones that are colorful and flavorful. But I like saran wrap because you can see through it. I wasn't perfect at safe sex at first and so I lived with anxiety afterward. I'd have post-orgasmic anxiety for weeks. Then as I got better at it, I didn't have those feelings anymore.

One of the reasons that I refer only to safer sex rather than safe sex is that it can be quite difficult to "do it" right. Condoms break; dental dams or saran wrap can slip. It's certainly better to try than not to try, but you have to realize that any time two people are having sex, there is some risk of passing on an STD. Martha spoke of the altered state that sex can bring on. If someone is on the verge of having an orgasm and they notice the condom has come off or the dental dam has slipped away, are they really going to stop and start over, particularly when they know that it might not be possible to become that aroused again? In such circumstances I think that more often than not, safe or safer sex is going to go out the window. If a couple is using alcohol or drugs, that will also lessen the chances that they will practice safer sex. So Martha is 100 percent right. You have to think about the consequences before you begin and do all you can to ensure that you remain safe.

Martha—Herpes slowed me down. It made me tell the other person what I had and it slowed them down. Thank God for herpes or I would have died of AIDS.

That's a silver lining that others who are not gay have mentioned too. But it will only work if you allow it to. If you go ahead and have unprotected sex, then you're leaving yourself open to catching another STD, and another, and maybe even HIV. That goes for gays and straights. So definitely use the excuse that you have a duty to tell potential partners that you have herpes to protect yourself against getting other diseases. It doesn't matter what it takes to get you to practice safer sex, it only matters that you actually do it.

Martha—I was an incest survivor and because of that I was very promiscuous. Herpes made me see that sex was not the way that I should be connecting with other people. Sex is great if done for the right motives. Herpes made me get real. I had to be vulnerable. Before I had herpes I had a lot of ego. Before herpes I could get by on my looks and after herpes I had to become vulnerable. What a wonderful thing to be like everybody else. I was no longer the queen bee, but a person among persons. Herpes was my great equalizer. And I learned that what's really important is not money, cars, or looks, but connecting with another human being in your heart and soul.

As I said earlier, the lessons to be learned from the gay people I contacted were not limited to gays but apply to people of every sexual orientation, and vice versa. Martha is a group leader in North Carolina and I'm sure she does a wonderful job because she has seen the truth about sex. I only wish more people could learn that truth before they catch an STD and have it forced upon them.

I'd like to make one last point. When AIDS first gained notice, far too many people looked at it as a "gay" disease, as if it had nothing to do with them. Of course, now it is spreading at a rapid rate among heterosexuals. Those early days of AIDS were an opportunity that too many people passed up. Rather than getting them to be more careful, all they did was look down on gays. For anyone reading this book who doesn't have herpes, I hope that instead of looking down on the people who do have it, you skip the "I told you so" and instead take every precaution not to become a statistic, of herpes or any other STD. These diseases are preventable, but only if everyone does their part.

Chapter Highlights

1. No STD is "cool."
2. Having herpes increases the risk of getting AIDS.
3. Even though support groups are mostly straight, they can still be helpful to gays.

12

Other STDs

From an early age, we teach our children to cover their mouths when they sneeze, bundle up when they go out into the cold, and wash their hands before dinner. Perhaps it's because they still catch colds that so many of them also ignore the advice we give them about safer sex practices when they become adults. People also engage in risky behavior because lust can overpower the rational side of our brains. When people are very aroused, they don't always listen to that little voice in their head telling them to be careful. Yet even though some people ignore the risks, many others do practice safer sex, and one would hope that people who've already been burned by one STD would be more likely to heed the cautionary warnings about the others.

Since I've now written an entire book on just one of these diseases, it's obvious I could write another one on all the others, if not a dozen or so. But while I'm not going to give you anywhere near that much information about the various STDs, I also don't want to miss this opportunity of giving you at least some cursory knowledge of some of the other diseases that are out there. I'm not going to go into every one because of space limitations, both in this book and in your brain. But given that you just read an entire book about herpes, I'm sure that if from what you read here you think that you're at risk for one of these other diseases, you'll go ahead and do more research on your own. And/or go straight to your doctor to be examined.

STDs have been around for a long time. Looking back at what records we have, we know they've existed for at least 3,500 years. But when you consider how widespread STDs are—they account for five out of ten common diseases reported to the Centers for Disease Control and Prevention—it's quite likely that they've been around much longer than that, though people back then didn't always recognize the cause. One reason for this is that the symptoms may not become apparent right away. For example, the red painless lesions that indicate the first signs of syphilis don't show themselves until at least three weeks after exposure. How likely is it that a primitive human would have made the connection between such a disease and intercourse with a particular person three weeks earlier?

But even though we've now made tremendous strides in science and medicine, we haven't been able to stop the spread of these diseases. Yes, in some cases we've found treatments and cures that never existed before, but many STDs are so widespread that they are considered to have reached epidemic proportions. So if you're having sex with multiple partners, the odds of running across one or more of these are pretty darn good. Yes, condoms can protect you, but condoms can break or fall off, so there's no such thing as safe sex, only safer sex.

In any case, here they are, the basic STDs. Since herpes is caused by a virus, I'm going to begin with the other STDs that are caused by viruses.

Human Papilloma Virus (HPV)

While HPV comes in different varieties—scientists have found more than one hundred—the form that most people know about causes genital warts. Altogether there are about thirty types of HPV that can be transmitted sexually, though most people don't realize they've been infected, and also don't realize the potential longer-term negative effects.

Many people who have HSV also have HPV. That's not surprising since HPV is so contagious and most people with herpes have been exposed to multiple partners. Roughly two out of every three individuals who have been sexually active will become infected with HPV. And as with herpes, many people don't know that they've been infected with HPV. Even those who have warts may not know as they can be microscopic in size, though others are quite visible and, shall we say, quite wartlike. But what HPV does to the appearance of your genitals isn't the main problem. Some types of HPV have been implicated in the development of cervical cancer, penile cancer, and anal cancer.

Though the warts themselves can be treated, the virus never leaves the infected person's body, and so even if the treatment is initially successful, the warts may come back. In many cases, the warts disappear on their own. If they grow and need to be treated, there are various therapies, some which require a doctor to apply and two of which are topical creams that may be applied by the patient. Small warts can also be removed by freezing them (cryosurgery) or may be burned off with a laser or electrocautery. Larger warts may require surgery.

Protecting Your Health

Because HPV infection of the genital area is transmitted by skin-to-skin contact, condoms offer some protection, but not 100 percent.

Certainly you should avoid any sexual contact with someone who has visible warts. However, HPV can be transmitted even in the absence of visible lesions. Even more important for women, if you have any suspicion that you may have been in contact with HPV, do not neglect your yearly Pap test. The biggest danger posed by HPV is the risk of cervical cancer, but if any irregular cells are spotted in time, the danger can be mitigated by early treatment.

Hepatitis

There are many types of hepatitis, starting with hepatitis A and going on up through the alphabet to G. Though hepatitis can be transferred in many ways, including the transmission of hepatitis B and C through sharing of needles by drug addicts, hepatitis A, B, and C may be passed on by the exchange of bodily fluids from vaginal intercourse or oral or anal sex. Although for some forms of hepatitis, namely hepatitis B, the virus is found in saliva, kissing is not likely to cause transmission.

In its initial stages, hepatitis causes symptoms such as nausea, dizziness, headache, abdominal pain, and fatigue, which could be caused by many diseases, but as the disease progresses it damages the liver, and up to 10,000 people die each year because of the damage done by one of the forms of hepatitis. There are an estimated 300,000 new cases of hepatitis B and 250,000 new cases of hepatitis C in this country each year. Because symptoms can be misread in a disease's early stages, it is important that a doctor perform a blood test to determine their actual cause. Obviously, the more risky behavior that a person indulges in, the greater the risks and so the greater the need of testing if any symptoms are felt.

Condoms provide some protection against hepatitis, and avoiding the sharing of certain personal hygiene products like toothbrushes and razors is also important. (College roommates and soldiers are groups that commonly fall victim to hepatitis.) Since 1982 there has been a vaccine against hepatitis B, and young children are now vaccinated as part of childhood vaccination or as a requirement for school entry. Effective vaccines are available for hepatitis A and are recommended for all men who have sex with men. There are treatments for people who come down with chronic viral hepatitis but they are expensive, require months of treatment, and are not 100 percent effective. Most episodes of acute hepatitis are treated with bed rest, proper diet, and the avoidance of alcohol.

HIV

When I first became "Dr. Ruth," that is to say, when my radio show began in 1980, no one outside the medical community had heard of AIDS yet. I would get many questions about herpes, and that disease even made the cover of *Time* magazine. But not long afterward it was discovered that the cause of the symptoms of so many young gay men was the human immunodeficiency virus (HIV), and from that moment on the very nature of sexual conduct was altered. Now there existed the risk of catching a life-threatening disease that had no cure, because of sexual contact. And while it was at first thought that this risk was limited to the homosexual community, or at least only those who practiced anal sex, sadly we've learned that people of all sexual orientations and who use any sexual position are at risk.

If untreated, HIV gradually destroys the body's capacity to combat certain infections and plays a role in the development of certain cancers. HIV can be in a person's body for a long time (as long as fifteen years) without causing AIDS and scientists are still unsure of why some individuals progress rapidly and others take a decade or longer to progress to AIDS.

HIV is what is known as a retrovirus. Once it enters a cell, it uses an enzyme to turn its RNA into DNA and actually becomes a part of the cell's genes. The virus then makes new parts (I'm simplifying here for brevity) that migrate into bodily fluids such as blood, semen, and vaginal and cervical fluids, and even mother's milk. When one of these body fluids containing these virus particles comes into contact with another person's mucosal membranes in the vagina, vulva, penis, rectum, or, some think, the mouth, the virus may enter the other person's bloodstream. If this person has any other STDs at this time, especially one involving open lesions as in syphilis or genital herpes, HIV more easily passes through the mucous membranes. Two weeks to a month after infection, many people will have what they think is a bad case of the flu. The body fights back, but the HIV can't be entirely eliminated. The average person begins to manifest the symptoms of AIDS about ten to twelve years after the initial infection. Some people, however, about 10 percent, will develop AIDS earlier, in as little as two to three years, while about 5 percent fail to develop AIDS even after twelve years. The amount of HIV in the bloodstream, called the *viral load,* is apparently an indicator of how rapid the progression of the disease will be.

Even though someone with HIV may show no symptoms for years, the HIV is multiplying in the lymphatic system. When the virus spills out of the lymphatic system into the bloodstream, the person becomes especially vulnerable to a number of different opportunistic infections. Literally billions of such particles are found in the bloodstream and because of mutations, they are not all identical, which is why finding one vaccine that will protect someone against all the variations is so difficult.

The Importance of Early Detection

Anyone who thinks that they may have been exposed to HIV shouldn't stick their head in the sand but should rush to be tested. The sooner that doctors can begin aggressive treatment, the more limited will be the amount of virus produced, which in turn will slow down disease progression and limit the development of opportunistic infections. An early diagnosis also allows one to inform any sexual partners so that they can be tested and benefit from the same early treatment.

There are a number of drugs that can slow down the replication of the virus. Since HIV can become resistant to them, they are typically used in combination, in a so-called cocktail. While these drugs may slow down the process, for now they cannot either eliminate HIV from a person's body or render someone noninfectious. These drugs also have many side effects, including nausea, diarrhea, and other gastrointestinal problems.

I've only scratched the surface of all there is to know about AIDS. Because it is so deadly and spreading so rapidly, it has attracted many research dollars and we have learned a lot about it. All you really need to know, however, is that as someone with herpes you are at greater risk to become infected by HIV than someone who does not have an STD, so that you must practice safer sex not only to prevent spreading herpes, but also to keep yourself from getting HIV. And, again, if you think you may have been infected, don't pretend that it will go away on its own, but instead go to see your doctor. The earlier you can detect the presence of HIV, the better you can fight off its effects.

STDs Caused by Bacteria

Bacteria arc huge compared to viruses, and instead of invading a cell to replicate, they do it on their own by dividing. The biggest difference between these two subsets of STDs is that because medical science has an effective way of reducing bacteria's ability to divide and multiply, the diseases caused by bacteria are easier to control. But this good news is mitigated by the fact that bacteria have "learned" to adapt and antibiotics that were once quite potent at stopping a particular STD no longer work. For example, one particular strain of gonorrhea not only became resistant to the antibiotic penicillin, but actually began to use the drug as a nutrient and grew actively in its presence! The drug companies have been working feverishly to catch up by creating new antibiotics to which disease-causing bacteria are not resistant, but it's a running battle and at this point we're not entirely sure who's ahead. Take this as one more reason to practice safer sex because even the STDs caused by bacteria, which were once easy to control, no longer are.

Chlamydia

The most common bacterial STD in the United States is chlamydia, with approximately three million new cases a year. Chlamydia is often a "silent" STD, as it may have no immediate symptoms. When symptoms do occur, they are more frequently seen in men and include a urethral discharge (pus coming out of the penis) and painful urination. In more serious cases, other parts of the body may swell and become painful, including the testicle and the prostate. Some women, about 15 percent, also have a discharge because of chlamydia, but most have no symptoms, though they are capable of passing on the disease. I should say no outward symptoms, because the biggest danger of chlamydia is that it can lead to pelvic inflammatory disease (PID), which can cause scarring of the fallopian tubes, which can make it difficult or impossible for a woman to become pregnant.

Condoms can help prevent the spread of this disease, and there are antibiotics that can cure chlamydia, but because so many people have it without symptoms, many physicians advise any person under the age of twenty-five who has had multiple sexual partners to be screened for chlamydia even if they are asymptomatic. That may save many women from discovering later in life that they are unable to conceive a child because they had an untreated case of chlamydia when they were younger.

Gonorrhea

Gonorrhea is the second most common bacterial STD in the United States. A slang name for gonorrhea is "the clap." Gonorrhea and chlamydia share some similarities in that they can cause a discharge but may also show no symptoms, especially in women. Most men will have a discharge and painful urination two to fourteen days after they have been infected. Like chlamydia, gonorrhea can cause PID, which can make a woman infertile, and it can also cause epididymitis in men, which can make a man infertile.

Gonorrhea can be treated with antibiotics, but there are more and more resistant strains cropping up, particularly in Asia. In China, for example, 70 percent of the cases of gonorrhea are resistant to the more common antibiotics. Another alarming statistic is that cases of rectal gonorrhea are on the rise among the homosexual population, which is an indicator that more homosexuals are not practicing safer sex by using condoms, and so are also at a greater risk of getting AIDS.

Syphilis

There is some debate as to how syphilis arrived in the Western world, with one theory having it brought back from the "New World" by Christopher Columbus, but whatever the reality, it did make its first appearance in Europe around that time and was a major scourge for centuries. If not treated, syphilis can be fatal, but the invention of penicillin made curing the disease very easy and greatly reduced the incidence of this STD in the United States. However, syphilis remains a danger because having sores caused by this disease can increase the risk of getting HIV.

Syphilis is caused by the bacterium *Treponema pallidium,* which looks like a little corkscrew. The STD goes through a num-

ber of different stages, each with its own symptoms and manifesta-
tions. The first, or primary, stage is characterized by a small ulcer
at the point where the bacteria first penetrated the skin or mucous
membrane; this is called a *chancre*. It usually appears two to six
weeks after exposure to the bacterium. The chancre causes no discomfort and in women it may be located inside the vagina, where
it would be hard to notice. If untreated, the chancre will disappear
on its own after a few weeks. The secondary stage is characterized
by a flat rash that may involve the palms and soles and may also be
characterized by small, round, white-colored skin sores that appear
three to six weeks after the chancre appears. These signs of infection may be accompanied by fatigue, headache, swollen lymph
nodes, and a sore throat. Each sore contains thousands of bacteria,
so any contact can readily transmit the disease. If untreated, these
sores will also disappear on their own, though they may recur a
number of times over a year or two.

If the disease has not been treated, it enters the latency stage.
Though the person is no longer contagious, the bacteria remains
inside the body. Two out of three people never get any symptoms
again. In those who develop tertiary syphilis, the bacteria can cause
damage to various internal organs, in particular the heart and brain,
as well as bones, joints, and eyes, which can lead to blindness, heart
attacks, stroke, dementia, and even death.

Condom use is very effective in protecting against syphilis,
since the primary stage chancre is usually located on the genitals.
However, it is important to have any genital lesion or growth examined by a doctor.* Taking a chance that syphilis won't enter the
tertiary stage is too big a risk.

*If one has been engaging in unprotected sexual intercourse and develops a rash
involving the palms and soles or has genital lesions accompanied with fever and
swollen lymph nodes, it is of utmost importance to be seen by a doctor.

Protect Yourself and Others

In this book we've seen how important it is to tell any potential partners if you have herpes, and we've also seen the benefits that can be derived from such honesty. The same philosophy must prevail when it comes to all the STDs I've mentioned, along with those I haven't. These diseases are almost all in epidemic proportions, both here and abroad. In cases where a person doesn't know that he or she is infected, no one is to blame. But far too often an infected person doesn't tell any sexual partners and ends up continuing the spread of whichever disease he or she may have. As we've seen in this book, it's not easy to tell someone you have an STD, but I've also given you help in how to do it, and that advice applies not just to herpes but also to any other STD.

So when it comes to STDs, the bottom line is that everyone should stick to the Golden Rule and be up front about any STD they may have. At the same time, you must all take great care to practice safer sex, not only to protect any partners, but also to protect yourself from any of the diseases that we've covered in this chapter.

Chapter Highlights

1. Sexually transmitted diseases exist in epidemic proportions in this country.
2. It's important to go to the doctor to be examined at the very first sign of any possible STD.
3. No matter which STD you may contract, you must work to protect any future partners.

Appendix A

The following support groups are the ones listed on the American Social Health Association (ASHA) website, which I've listed here for those of you who don't have computer access. For those readers with computer access, you can find some additional groups listed in the Social and Support Networking Alliance, whose website is listed in Appendix B.

Local HELP (Support) Groups

Arizona

Phoenix Valley HELP
Phoenix, AZ
(602) 867-6613
Web: *http://valleyhelp.hypermart.net*

California

Los Angeles HELP
Culver City, CA
(310) 281-7511
Web: *http://www.lahelp.org*

Northern California HELP
c/o Solano Clinical Research
2 Groups—Vallejo and Davis
(707) 643-5785 (Vallejo)
(530) 757-7797 (Davis)
E-mail: *research@solderm.com*

Orange County HELP
Orange, CA
(949) 753-2580
Web: *http://www.lahelp.org/index2.htm*

San Diego City HELP
San Diego, CA
(619) 491-1194
E-mail: *pitcairn@rohan.sdsu.edu*
Web: *http://www.aznet.net/~pitcairn/herpes/support.html*

San Francisco HELP
San Francisco, CA
(415) 664-5078

South Bay HELP
Mountain View, CA
(408) 296-1444

Connecticut

Fairfield & Westchester Co. HELP
c/o HealthGain
(203) 975-2451
E-mail: *fbtworld@aol.com*

Manchester HELP
Manchester, CT
(860) 445-5863 (Annie)
(860) 666-0075 (Susan)
E-mail: *hsv2secret@aol.com*

Delaware

HELP of Delaware
c/o Omega Medical Center
Newark, DE
(302) 368-9625

District of Columbia

HELP of Washington
Washington, DC
(301) 369-1323
Web: *http://www.herpeshelpofwashington.org*

Florida

Broward and Palm Beach HELP
Coral Springs, FL
(954) 896-9788
E-mail: *helpinsfl@yahoo.com*

Central Florida HELP
Orlando, FL
(407) 263-5347
Web: *http://www.geocities.com/orlandohelpgroup*

Tampa Bay HELP
2 Groups—Tampa and Clearwater
(813) 677-1633

Georgia

Atlanta HELP
Atlanta, GA
(404) 294-6364

Illinois

Chicago HELP
Chicago, IL
(773) 660-0416
E-mail: *info@chicagohelp.org*
Web: *http://www.chicagohelp.org*

Indiana

Fort Wayne HELP
c/o Park Center, Inc.
Fort Wayne, IN
(260) 481-2890
E-mail: *ftwaynehelp@ftwaynehelp-hpv.com*
Web: *http://www.ftwaynehelp-hpv.com*

Indy HELP
Indianapolis, IN
(317) 221-8313
E-mail: *IndyHelp@yahoo.com*
Web: *http://www.indyhelp.com*

Southern Indiana HELP
Shirley, IN
(765) 785-9219
E-mail: *gayla@hrtc.net*

Kentucky

Kentuckiana HELP
Louisville, KY
(502) 380-9122
E-mail: *kirvin2@yahoo.com*

Lousiana

New Orleans HELP
Metairie, LA
(504) 733-5104

Maine

Maine HELP
c/o City of Bangor STD Clinic
Bangor, ME
(207) 947-0700

Massachusetts

Boston HELP
Boston, MA
(781) 648-4266
E-mail: *bostonhelp@mail.racoon.com*
Web: *http://www.bostonherpes.org*

Michigan

Grand Rapids HELP
Holland, MI
(616) 252-4900

Metro Detroit HELP
Eastpointe, MI
(586) 447-2699
E-mail: *info@metrodetroithelp.org*
Web: *http://www.metrodetroithelp.org*

Traverse City HELP
Traverse City, MI
(800) 442-7315 (toll-free)
E-mail: *monkey_method@hotmail.com*

Washtenaw County HELP
Novi, MI
(248) 788-5816
E-mail: *help@annarborhelp.org*
Web: *http://www.annarborhelp.org*

Minnesota

Twin Cities HELP
Minneapolis-St. Paul, MN
(800) 78-FACTS (toll-free MN only)

Missouri

Kansas City HELP
Kansas City, MO
(913) 599-9715
Web: *http://hometown.aol.com/Ihaveittoo/index.html*

Ozarks HELP
Springfield, MO
(417) 875-6424
Web: *http://www.ozarkshelp.com*

St. Louis "SHEPH" HELP
St. Louis, MO
(636) 230-2288
E-mail: *stl_sheph@yahoo.com*

Nebraska

Omaha HELP
Omaha, NE
(402) 895-1484
E-mail: *yoshi2me@cox.net*
Web:*http://members.cox.net/yoshi2me/OmahaHELP/*
   OmahaHELPx.html

New Jersey

Central New Jersey HELP
Toms River, NJ
(732) 270-4680
E-mail: *CNJ_HELP@yahoo.com*
Web: *http://geocities.com/cnj_help/ginaz.html*

South Jersey HELP
Pleasantville, NJ
(609) 748-6239
(609) 748-2518
E-mail: *HCIR@netzero.net*
E-mail: *smilingrl43@aol.com*
Web: *http://www.geocities.com/moonlite7us/SJerseyHELP.html*

New York

Long Island HELP
Plainview, NY
(631) 361-9338
E-mail: *ocean@racoon.com*

New York HELP
New York, NY
(212) 628-9154
E-mail: *help@nyhelp.org*
Web: *http://www.nyhelp.org*

North Carolina

Capital HELP
c/o Planned Parenthood
Raleigh, NC
(919) 833-7534
Web: *http://www.plannedparenthood.org/ppcc*

Charlotte HELP
c/o Carolina Women's Clinic
Charlotte, NC
(704) 556-6838

Coastal HELP
c/o Planned Parenthood
Wilmington, NC
(910) 762-5566
Web: *http://www.plannedparenthood.org/ppcc*

Mountain HELP
Asheville, NC
(828) 669-5188
E-mail: *mtnhelp@juno.com*

Triad HELP
c/o Guilford Co. Dept. of Public Health
and Planned Parenthood of Greensboro, NC
(336) 641-4699

Wayne County HELP
Goldsboro, NC
(919) 739-0076
E-mail: *wayne_co_help@yahoo.com*

Ohio

Cincinnati HELP
Cincinnati, OH
(513) 557-3435
E-mail: *cincinnati_help@yahoo.com*
Web: *http://www.cincinnatihelp.org/*

Cleveland HELP
Cleveland, OH
(216) 556-2817
E-mail: *cleh2@aol.com*
Web: *http://www.geocities.com/cleH2/*

Columbus HELP
Columbus, OH
(614) 470-0709
E-mail: *columbushelp@yahoo.com*
Web: *http://www.columbushelp.4t.com*

Dayton HELP
c/o Wright State University—Ellis Institute
Dayton, OH
(937) 775-4300

Oklahoma

Tulsa HELP
c/o Planned Parenthood
Tulsa, OK
(918) 587-1101
E-mail: *WeHELPinTulsa@yahoo.com*
Web: *http://www.geocities.com/wehelpintulsa/TulsaHELP.html*

Oregon

Portland Area HELP
Portland, OR
(503) 727-2640
E-mail: *portlandareahelp@aol.com*

Pennsylvania

Philadelphia HELP
Philadelphia, PA
(610) 896-9601
E-mail: *Philly437@hotmail.com*

Tri State HELP
Pittsburgh, PA
(412) 341-8920
E-mail: *Jbretz3452@aol.com*

Rhode Island

Providence HELP
c/o Family Services, Inc.
Providence, RI
(401) 331-1350

South Carolina

Columbia HELP
Columbia, SC
(803) 781-5280
E-mail: *info@columbiahelp.com*
Web: *http://www.columbiahelp.com*

Texas

Austin HELP
Austin, TX
(512) 247-5551
E-mail: *support@austinhelp.org*
Web: *http://www.austinhelp.org*

Fort Worth HELP
c/o Planned Parenthood
Fort Worth, TX
(817) 882-1155

Frontera HELP
c/o Planned Parenthood
Harlingen, TX
(956) 425-7526

Houston HELP
Houston, TX
(866) 841-9139 x 2551 (toll-free)
E-mail: *HoustonHELP@yahoo.com*
Web: *http://www.houstonhelp.org*

San Antonio HELP
c/o Planned Parenthood
San Antonio, TX
(210) 989-0104

Virginia

Richmond HELP
c/o Fan Free Clinic
Richmond, VA
(804) 358-6343

Washington

Seattle HELP
Seattle, WA
(206) 726-4478

West Virginia

Northcentral West Virginia HELP
c/o West Virginia University
Morgantown, WV
(304) 293-6972

Canada

Alberta

Calgary HELP
Calgary, AB
(403) 228-7400

British Columbia

Vancouver HELP
Vancouver, BC
(604) 515-5500
Web: *http://groups.yahoo.com/group/vancouverhelp/*

Manitoba

Winnipeg HELP
Winnipeg, MB
(204) 940-2200

Ontario

Toronto HELP
c/o The Phoenix Association
Toronto, ON
(416) 449-0876
E-mail: *phoenix_association@hotmail.com*
Web: *http://www.torontoherpes.com*

Quebec

Montreal HELP
St. Laurent, QC
(514) 855-8995
E-mail: *ruban-en-route@qc.aira.com*
Web: *http://www.rubanenroute.org/herpes.php*

Appendix B

Web References

www.ashastd.org—The American Social Health Association is dedicated to improving the health of individuals, families, and communities, with a focus on preventing the transmission of sexually transmitted diseases and their harmful consequences. This site includes facts and answers, chat rooms, and other resources.

www.cdc.gov—The Centers for Disease Control and Prevention, the main public health agency of the U.S. government, has information on just about every disease, including herpes. When looking up herpes in the *A* to *Z* index, make sure you look up genital herpes under *G*, not herpes under *H*.

www.niaid.nih.gov—The National Institute of Allergy and Infectious Diseases (NIAID) is a component of the National Institutes of Health (NIH). NIAID conducts and supports research that strives to understand, treat, and ultimately prevent the myriad infectious, immunologic, and allergic diseases that threaten hundreds of millions of people worldwide. Their fact sheets are constantly updated.

www.herpeshelp.com—This site is run by GlaxoSmithKline, the makers of the drug valacyclovir (Valtrex), and contains much useful information about herpes in general.

www.genitalherpes.com—This site is run by Novartis, the drug company that makes famciclovir (Famvir), and contains much useful information about herpes in general.

www.herpes.org—This site is run by a doctor, who calls himself Dr. H. Many of the people I spoke with for this book use this site to get information.

http://www.yoshi2me.com—Social and Support Networking Alliance is a site that was put together by people with herpes, including some of whom I spoke with for this book. It has a more detailed list of support groups than the one put together by ASHA which I used for Appendix A (though the information on how to reach them is "clickable," so that you must use a computer to access it), and lots of other links. You can find personal stories, get on the herpes web ring, and find message boards.

www.goaskalice.columbia.edu—This site is run by Columbia University and does a very good job of answering questions about all sorts of issues dealing with sexuality, not just STDs.

www.drruth.com—This will take you to my area on iVIllage.com. I don't have much material on herpes, but if you register for the message boards, you can ask questions, some of which I answer, but also many of which draw responses from other readers, many of whom give useful advice. These are many about relationships, but that's what this book is really about too, so if you have a relationship problem, why not try our boards out.

Index